Oral
Medicine

A Pocket Guide

Oral Medicine
A Pocket Guide

Lewis R. Eversole, D.D.S., M.S.D., M.A.
Professor
Section of Diagnostic Sciences and Facial Pain
School of Dentistry
University of California at Los Angeles Medical Center
Los Angeles, California

W.B. SAUNDERS COMPANY
A Division of Harcourt Brace & Company
Philadelphia   London   Toronto   Montreal   Sydney   Tokyo

W.B. Saunders Company
A Division of Harcourt Brace & Company

The Curtis Center
Independence Square West
Philadelphia, Pennsylvania 19106

Library of Congress Cataloging-in-Publication Data

Eversole, Lewis R.
    Oral medicine: a pocket guide   /   Lewis R. Eversole.—
1st ed.
      p.   cm.
    ISBN 0–7216–4973–4
    1. Oral medicine–Handbooks, manuals, etc.   I. Title.
    [DNLM: 1. Mouth Diseases–drug therapy–handbooks.   WU 49 E93o
1996]
RC815.E96   1996
617.5′22—dc20
DNLM/DLC   94–47441

Oral Medicine: A Pocket Guide   ISBN 0–7216–4973–4

Printed in the United States of America.

Last digit is the print number: 9   8   7   6   5   4   3   2

*Dedicated to
all dental students and residents
who work so hard to achieve their goals
to become competent and caring
health care providers.*

PREFACE

Oral medicine is a discipline that subsumes internal medicine as it impacts on dental care; management of medically ill patients; diagnosis of systemic disease on the basis of oral, head, and neck manifestations; diagnosis and management of oral soft tissue diseases; and diagnosis and management of facial pain. Many textbooks are available to the student that detail the concepts of physical diagnosis, internal medicine, oral medicine, oral pathology, and differential diagnosis, and such texts are reliable, essential reference sources. In the clinic setting, many decisions must be made on a variety of fronts, including assessment of a patient's medical status, the drugs that have to be prescribed for them, and precautions that must be taken to ensure safe dental management. This is of particular concern in an aging society. Additionally, signs and symptoms of oral disease must be assessed, and decisions must be made to arrive at a definitive diagnosis and render appropriate care. *Oral Medicine: A Pocket Guide* has been designed to meet the needs of the clinician in the area of diagnosis and patient management. The text is concise and to the point, providing the appropriate guidelines for managing oral medicine problems that will be confronted by the generalist and various specialists in dentistry.

LEWIS R. EVERSOLE, D.D.S., M.S.D., M.A.

CONTENTS

Dental Implications of Medical Conditions

Cardiovascular and Renal Diseases

HYPERTENSION

Etiology

Stress—benign, essential
Arteriolosclerosis—malignant

Consequences for Dental Care

Stroke
Angina attack
Myocardial infarction

Causes of Consequences

Dental fear and anxiety predispose to catecholamine release with hypertensive crisis and tachycardia, which can induce angina, myocardial infarction, or cerebrovascular accident, the last being most probable.

Management

1. Ensure that blood pressure is controlled by medication to a diastolic level below 100 mm Hg before initiating any type of dental care.
2. Use local anesthetic with vasoconstrictor to be sure that anesthesia is adequate. Refraining from vasoconstrictor use can result in inadequate anesthesia, pain, anxiety, and an episode of hypertension or tachycardia related to the release of endogenous catecholamines. For diastolic pressures over 100, vasoconstrictors may be withheld.
3. When using anesthesia with vasoconstrictor, always aspirate before injection and do not use more than four cartridges.
4. Never use epinephrine-soaked retraction cord for impressions in hypertensive patients.

Oral Manifestations

None

VASCULAR OCCLUSIVE DISEASE

Etiology

Hyperlipidemia—atherosclerosis
High-fat diet
Familial deficiency of lipid receptors for apoproteins

Consequences for Dental Care

Acute: Patients may experience angina or develop myocardial infarction or cerebrovascular accident intraoperatively.

Chronic: Medication used to treat vascular disease can cause problems:
  1. Antihypertensive agents, diuretics—xerostomia
  2. Anticoagulants—hemorrhagic diathesis

Postinfarction arrhythmias may be managed with pacemakers.

Causes of Consequences

1. Arterial plaque
   a. Myocardial infarction
   b. Cerebrovascular accident
   c. Aortic aneurysm
   d. Carotid aneurysm
2. Venous plaque
   a. Thrombophlebitis—pulmonary embolus

Management

1. Assess coagulation level if the patient is on anticoagulant therapy. Normal prothrombin time is 11 to 15 seconds; do not perform any procedure that may cause bleeding if this value is twice normal.
2. Review CPR life support before appointment. Make sure the patient brings all vasodilators, and place them close by. Monitor vital signs.
3. Xerostomia can predispose to tooth decay and is annoying to patients. Discuss with physician possibility of changing to a less xerostomatogenic drug.
4. Pacemakers can be altered by ultrasonic cleaning equipment and scalers.
5. Assess stress level. Shorten appointments or prescribe an anxiolytic medication if necessary.

Oral Manifestations

Left mandibular pain in angina and myocardial infarction

CONGENITAL HEART DISEASE

Etiology

Birth defects in development of heart chambers and valves with abnormal heart sounds and murmurs

Complications

Congestive heart failure

Bacterial endocarditis or endarteritis
Polycythemia with thrombocytopenia in patients with shunts

Consequences for Dental Care

Dyspnea or breathing difficulty when reclined
Inhalation anesthesia risk
Oral bacteremia
Excessive bleeding

Causes of Consequences

1. Valvular stenosis or insufficiency
2. Aortic coarctation
3. Atrial and ventricular septal defects
4. Patent ductus arteriosus
5. Transposition of the great vessels
6. Eisenmenger's complex
7. Tetralogy of Fallot

Management

1. Review vital signs, particularly heart rate. If the patient has severe tachycardia, discuss possibility of heart failure with physician.
2. If signs of congestive heart failure are observed, do not recline the patient for prolonged periods; periodically check vital signs.
3. Review CPR life support before appointment.
4. Monitor platelet count in patients with atrial or ventricular shunts.
5. Prophylactic antibiotics are required in all cases in which surgical correction of the heart defect has not been undertaken.

Oral Manifestations

None

RHEUMATIC HEART DISEASE

Etiology

Poststreptococcal (rheumatic fever) immunopathologic tissue inflammation and scarring

Consequences for Dental Care

Bacterial endocarditis
Arrhythmia—pacemaker
Congestive heart failure

Causes of Consequences

1. Aseptic vegetative valvulitis with murmur
2. Myocardial inflammatory foci interfering with conduction
3. Inadequate cardiac output

Management

1. Use prophylactic antibiotics.
2. Review vital signs, particularly heart rate. If the patient has severe tachycardia, discuss possibility of heart failure with physician.
3. If signs of congestive failure are observed, do not recline the patient for prolonged periods; periodically check vital signs.
4. Review CPR life support before appointment.
5. Follow precautions for pacemaker if present.

Oral Manifestations

None

VALVULAR DISEASE

Etiology

Rheumatic heart disease
Congenital stenosis or insufficiency
Mitral valve prolapse with regurgitation
Surgical correction—prosthetic valve

Consequences for Dental Care

Bacterial endocarditis
Congestive heart failure

Causes of Consequences

1. Turbulent flow around damaged valve leads to endocarditis following dental procedures that result in bacteremia.
2. Cardiac output becomes decreased, leading to heart failure.

Management

1. Use prophylactic antibiotics.
2. Review vital signs, particularly heart rate. If the patient has severe tachycardia, discuss possibility of heart failure with physician.
3. If signs of congestive failure are observed, do not recline the patient for prolonged periods; periodically check vital signs.
4. Review CPR life support before appointment.

Oral Manifestations

None

PROSTHETIC VALVE

Etiology

Valvular stenosis or insufficiency of such severity that surgical valve replacement became necessary

Consequences for Dental Care

Bacterial endocarditis
Congestive heart failure

Causes of Consequences

1. Prosthesis, whether metal or biological (animal) tissue, becomes subject to bacterial colonization after dental procedures that cause bacteremia.
2. Prosthesis may not completely correct pre-existing cardiac failure.

Management

1. Use prophylactic antibiotics.
2. Review vital signs, particularly heart rate. If the patient has severe tachycardia, discuss possibility of heart failure with physician.
3. If signs of congestive failure are observed, do not recline the patient for prolonged periods; periodically check vital signs.
4. Review CPR life support before appointment.

Oral Manifestations

None

BACTERIAL ENDOCARDITIS

Etiology

Streptococci of oral origin
Genitourinary tract microbes

Consequence for Dental Care

Endocarditis

Cause of Consequence

A history of endocarditis implies that endocardial damage is present and that the process could occur again given a new bacteremia

Management

Administer prophylactic antibiotics before any procedure that causes oral bleeding.

Oral Manifestations

None

ARRHYTHMIA AND PACEMAKER USE

Etiology

Conduction defects
    From myocardial infarction
    Postrheumatic myocarditis
    Acidosis
    Drug-induced
Pacemaker

Consequences for Dental Care

Cardiogenic shock
Cardiac arrest

Causes of Consequences

1. Interference with cardiac conduction pathways can result from necrosis or inflammation involving conduction fibers leading to irregular heart rhythm or fibrillation. Additional stress in dental office or dental pain could induce tachycardia or disturb any coexisting cardiovascular problems (e.g., valvular disease, coronary artery disease with congestive failure).
2. Cardiac arrest could evolve through electrical interference with a pacemaker.

Management

1. For surgery in an anxious patient with an arrhythmia, anxiolytic medication can be prescribed just before the appointment.
2. Monitor vital signs throughout procedures.
3. Use vasoconstrictor, 1 : 100,000 epinephrine in anesthetic, always aspirating. Never administer more than four cartridges. In extreme or severe arrhythmias, vasoconstrictor may be elimi-

nated from local anesthetic. To avoid adrenaline rush induced by pain from incomplete anesthesia, consider hospitalization with intravenous sedation or general anesthesia and cardiovascular monitoring.
4. Never use epinephrine-soaked retraction cord for crown impressions.
5. In patients with pacemakers, avoid ultrasonic cleaners and scalers as well as electronic pulp testers and electrosurgical units, since they can interfere with pacemaker signals.

Oral Manifestations

None

RENAL FAILURE AND HEMODIALYSIS

Etiology

Immune or infectious processes
Glomerulonephritis, pyelonephritis, tubular disease with uremia or nephrosis
Hemodialysis

Consequences for Dental Care

Bleeding tendency
Infected dialysis shunt
High-risk hepatitis B virus carrier

Causes of Consequences

1. Patients receive heparin for hemodialysis, and the anticoagulant effect persists for up to 6 hours.
2. Arteriovenous shunts for periodic insertion of dialysis needle can become infected (endarteritis) subsequent to bacteremia.

Management

1. Evaluate coagulation status. Delay dental procedures for 1 day after dialysis. Partial thromboplastin time may be ordered; do not undertake any oral surgical procedures if value is two times control levels.
2. Use antibiotic prophylaxis to prevent endarteritis in patients with shunts.
3. Use appropriate precautions for hepatitis infection risk.

Oral Manifestations

None

Immunocompromise and Autoimmune Diseases

ACQUIRED IMMUNODEFICIENCY SYNDROME (AIDS)

Etiology

Human immunodeficiency virus with depletion of CD4 helper lymphocytes, leading to infections and malignancies

Consequences for Dental Care

Bleeding tendency
Breathing difficulty
Inhalation anesthesia risk

Causes of Consequences

1. Some patients with AIDS experience idiopathic thrombocytopenic purpura.
2. Dyspnea evolves as a consequence of chronic *Pneumocystis* pneumonia and may pose a risk for inhalation anesthesia.

Management

1. Before any oral surgery, a platelet count should be obtained. Do not perform surgery if count is below 50,000. The procedure should be done in the hospital if a dental emergency exists so that platelets can be infused.
2. Do not prescribe aspirin-related analgesics for orodental pain if platelet count is low. Use acetaminophen, ibuprofen, codeine, or a combination.
3. If the patient is dyspneic, do not recline for long periods; monitor vital signs. If inhalation anesthesia is to be used, evaluate respiratory status.
4. Oral lesions should be definitively diagnosed by smear or biopsy, and appropriate treatment rendered. Bacterial odontogenic and periodontal infections are not a problem.
5. Severely ill patients should be hospitalized for oral surgery.

Oral Manifestations

Kaposi's sarcoma
Lymphoma
Oral infections
      Candida
      Hairy leukoplakia
      Invasive fungi

CANCER AND CHEMOTHERAPY

Etiology

Malignant neoplasia (solid tumors) of various organs
Breast adenocarcinoma
Bronchogenic carcinoma
Colon carcinoma
Thyroid carcinoma
Uterine cervix carcinoma
Lymphoma

Consequences for Dental Care

Delayed wound healing in the mouth
Bleeding tendency

Causes of Consequences

1. Overdose of chemotherapy inhibits bone marrow, with anemia, agranulocytosis, leukopenia, and thrombocytopenia.
2. Disseminated intravascular coagulation occurs in widespread cancer, leading to a consumptive coagulopathy.

Management

1. If ulcers are present, the patient is probably granulocytopenic and could die in a matter of days. Order complete blood count, and refer to treating physician.
2. If history or signs indicate a bleeding tendency, order complete blood count, platelet count, and partial thromboplastin time. If clotting values exceed twice control values or if platelet count is under 50,000, withhold surgery or admit the patient to the hospital for the procedure.
3. Do not prescribe aspirin-related analgesics for orodental pain if platelet count is low. Use acetaminophen, ibuprofen, codeine, or a combination.

Oral Manifestation

Oral ulcerations
Candidiasis

BONE MARROW TRANSPLANTATION

Etiology

Refractory leukemia, total body irradiation/chemotherapy—marrow HLA-matched allogeneic graft

Induced immunosuppression
Solid tumor, lymphoma, total body irradiation/chemotherapy—pretreatment autogenous graft

Consequences for Dental Care

Susceptibility to oral infections

Causes of Consequences

1. Patients with both allografts and autografts develop graft-versus-host disease (GVHD) and are therefore medicated to induce low-level immunosuppression. Immunoglobulin and T-cell functions are depressed. Oral herpes and bacterial infections can become severe and disseminated.
2. Autoimmune GVHD can result in the rejection phenomenon of oral mucosa causing a burning lichenoid stomatitis. Although uncommon, even autogenous grafts can induce GVHD.

Management

1. Ideally, the patient should have any oral disease treated before undergoing transplantation.
2. For odontogenic and periodontal infections, particularly those with purulence, medicate the patient with antibiotics, generally penicillin-related drugs. Usually, intravenous administration should be started, the dental problem treated, then the patient placed on oral antibiotic therapy. Oral sepsis should be kept to an absolute minimum in patients with bone marrow transplants.
3. Oral herpes lesions should be treated with systemically administered acyclovir; candidal infections are treated with antifungals.
4. Oral GVHD is a marker of more widespread rejection disease. Notify the patient's physician, since the immunosuppressive medication dosage may need to be increased.

Oral Manifestation

GVHD lichenoid stomatitis
Nonspecific stomatitis

ORGAN TRANSPLANTATION

Etiology

Organ failure
Kidney—nephritis
Heart—congestive failure
Heart/lung—congestive heart failure
Liver—cirrhosis
Allograft organ with induced immunosuppression

Consequences for Dental Care

Susceptibility to odontogenic infection
Susceptibility to viral and fungal oral infections

Cause of Consequences

Immunosuppressive medication lowers host resistance to infection
by debilitating immunoglobulin production and T-cell function.

Management

1. Ideally, the patient should have oral disease treated before transplantation.
2. If dental treatment is required during first 6 months after surgery, prescribe prophylactic antibiotics, usually penicillin-related drugs.
3. For odontogenic and periodontal infections, particularly those with purulence, medicate with antibiotics, generally penicillin-related drugs. Usually intravenous administration should be started, the dental problem treated, then the patient placed on oral antibiotic therapy. Oral sepsis should be kept to an absolute minimum in patients with transplants.
4. Oral herpes lesions should be treated with systemically administered acyclovir; candidal infections are treated with topical antifungals.

Oral Manifestations

Herpetic stomatitis
Candidiasis

HEAD AND NECK CANCER AND RADIATION THERAPY

Etiology

Cancer—tobacco, alcohol, papillomavirus
Radiation—affects on salivary glands and bone

Consequences for Dental Care

Xerostomia
Dental caries
Osteoradionecrosis

Causes of Consequences

1. Ablation of salivary parenchyma, leading to sclerosis of parotid and submandibular glands.
2. Radiation damage to intraosseous vasculature, preventing adequate vascularization of inflammatory tissue if osteomyelitis

occurs. Infection then leads to widespread necrosis and sequestration of bone.

Management

1. Dental consultation should be rendered before radiation therapy to remove all sources of sepsis.
2. Prescribe artificial saliva (e.g., Xero-Lube, lemon glycerin water).
3. Advise rigid daily fluoride applications to decrease caries incidence.
4. Advise chlorhexidine rinses to decrease periodontal pathogens and *Candida.*
5. Prescribe antifungal agents if candidiasis is present.
6. Remove all sources of infection that could lead to osteomyelitis (pulpal or periodontal infections).

Oral Manifestations

Radiation mucositis
Erythematous candidiasis
Root caries
Osteoradionecrosis

LUPUS ERYTHEMATOSUS

Etiology

Unknown—autoimmune collagen disease with autoantibodies to nucleic acids and histones

Consequences for Dental Care

Treatment with immunosuppressive drugs—susceptibility to oral infections
Painful oral lesions

Causes of Consequences

1. Immunosuppressive therapy may be necessary to treat more severe cases of lupus erythematosus (i.e., the systemic form is associated with glomerulonephritis and inflammatory joint disease). High steroid levels may predispose to oral infections.
2. Both the discoid and systemic types of lupus erythematosus involve the skin, and similar lesions can occur in the oral cavity, representing autoimmune lesions.

Management

1. Monitor the patient's level of steroid intake. Levels equivalent to over 40 mg of prednisone per day may predispose to oral infections,

particularly candidiasis. Odontogenic and periodontal infections may become worse or prolonged when the patient is on high steroid levels. In such cases, decreasing the steroids is advisable, as is prescription of the appropriate antibiotic.

2. Oral lesions that are manifestations of lupus erythematosus can be treated with topical steroid gels.

Oral Manifestations

Candidiasis associated with immunosuppression
Prolonged odontogenic infections associated with immunosuppression
Oral red, white, and erosive lesions of lupus erythematosus

SCLERODERMA

Etiology

Unknown—autoimmune disease causing collagenization of the skin and mucosa

Consequences for Dental Care

Microstomia
Affected gingival and oral tissues
Immunosuppressive drug use
Salivary involvement—secondary Sjögren syndrome

Causes of Consequences

1. The connective tissues underlying the cutaneous and mucosal epithelia become progressively collagenized, loosing pliability and becoming rigid.
2. Salivary acini are replaced by connective tissues, leading to xerostomia.
3. Other associated autoimmune disorders may occur including the CREST syndrome, arthritis, nephritis, and lupus.

Management

1. Many physicians recommend no treatment. Plasmaphoresis to remove immune complexes from the circulation benefits some patients. When other manifestations of collagen disease evolve, steroid therapy can be instituted.
2. Routine dental care is difficult because of a progressive decrease in the oral aperture. It is advisable to implement a thorough preventive maintenance program and to accomplish as much definitive dental care as possible while the patient is still able to open the mouth.

3. Close periodontal monitoring is necessary, and mucogingival strictures should be relieved surgically.

Oral Manifestations

Microstomia with limited opening, which is a problem for dental care

Mucogingival problems due to frenal pulls from fibrous strictures

MULTIPLE SCLEROSIS

Etiology

Autoimmune antibodies to myelin sheath proteins

Consequences for Dental Care

Facial neuropathies
Drug treatment—steroids

Causes of Consequences

1. Loss of myelin sheath from both sensory and motor nerves and perineural inflammatory changes can cause sensory deficits of the trigeminal nerve. These are usually in the form of hypoesthesia or paresthesia, although trigeminal neuralgia may occasionally be a complication. Seventh, fifth, or twelfth nerve involvement may be seen with attending motor weakness of the facial, masticatory, or intrinsic tongue muscles, respectively.

2. Steroid drug therapy can be a cause for concern if the dosage is high. There is a susceptibility to infection, especially oral candidiasis. Endodontic infections may become more widespread and acute.

Management

1. Assure patient that any facial neurologic problems are associated with multiple sclerosis and are not due to a dental or periodontal infection. Carbamazepine therapy may be indicated.

2. Stop antibiotic and drug therapy if high-dose steroids result in oral infectious disease.

Oral Manifestation

Facial neurologic deficits

Hepatic and Gastrointestinal Diseases

HEPATITIS

Etiology

Viral hepatitis A virus, hepatitis B virus, non-A, non-B (hepatitis C) virus, delta agent, hepatitis E

Epstein-Barr virus or mononucleosis
Nonviral (chemical) agents

Consequences for Dental Care

Disease transmission
Bleeding diathesis

Causes of Consequences

1. All viral types are contagious by blood transmission during active infection; hepatitis B virus and non-A, non-B virus exist in chronic as well as asymptomatic carrier states.
2. During active disease, when bilirubin and liver enzymes are elevated, and in postinfectious cirrhosis, liver failure results in deficiencies of clotting factors.

Management

1. If all staff have been vaccinated, office risk is eliminated. To prevent transmission to other patients, all equipment used on the patient must be sterilized with strict adherence to infection control procedures.
2. Any oral surgery procedures should await a work-up for disease status: hepatitis B virus C and E antigens connote infectivity; bilirubin and liver enzymes indicate status of infection; partial thromboplastin time assesses coagulation status. If partial thromboplastin time is more than twice control, the patient must be hospitalized for oral surgery.
3. Do not prescribe aspirin-related analgesics for orodental pain. Use acetaminophen, ibuprofen, codeine, or a combination.

Oral Manifestations

Purpura
Jaundice

CIRRHOSIS

Etiology

Alcoholism—Laënnec's cirrhosis
Cholelithiasis, pancreatic tumor, bile duct atresia—biliary origin
Hepatitis—postinfectious scarring
Drug-induced—chloroform, halothane

Consequences for Dental Care

Bleeding diathesis
Impaired drug metabolism

Causes of Consequences

1. Production of clotting factors by hepatocytes is decreased.
2. In biliary cirrhosis, malabsorption of fats leads to steatorrhea with fat-soluble vitamin deficiency, vitamin K in particular, compounding clotting deficiency.
3. Loss of hepatocytes leads to inability to clear certain drugs from circulation.

Management

1. Obtain prothrombin time (extrinsic pathway)—11 to 15 seconds are normal; partial thromboplastin time (intrinsic pathway)—25 to 35 seconds are normal. If these values exceed twice control values, do not undertake oral surgery or periodontal scaling. The patient should be hospitalized for such procedures so that missing factors can be administered.
2. Do not prescribe aspirin-related analgesics for orodental pain. Use acetaminophen, ibuprofen, codeine, or a combination.
3. Review drugs to be prescribed for prolonged effect, especially sedatives and analgesics. Lower the usual dosage.

Oral Manifestation

Ecchymosis

ANOREXIA NERVOSA AND BULIMIA

Etiology

Psychiatric eating disorders often associated with history of abuse

Consequences for Dental Care

Severe lingual dental erosion

Causes of Consequences

Forced vomiting after eating results in a constant bathing of the oral tissues with gastric acids that resorb tooth structure. If bulimic behavior has been taking place for many years, severe erosion may be seen.

Management

1. The patient should be informed of the loss of tooth structure and referred to a therapist or eating disorder clinic. Bulimic patients are often secretive about their disorder, and dental findings may be the first sign that the patient is suffering from psychiatric illness.

2. Lost tooth structure can be restored by laminates, cast gold, or bonded resins.

Oral Manifestation

Erosion of the lingual and palatal sufaces of enamel and eventually dentin
Parotid enlargement

GLUTEN ENTEROPATHY (Celiac Disease)

Etiology

Intestinal allergy to gliadin

Consequences for Dental Care

Associated oral lesions
Bleeding diathesis

Causes of Consequences

1. Hypersensitivity to gliadin found in various foodstuffs (grains) is often associated with oral ulcers.
2. Loss of intestinal villi leads to malabsorption, with resultant hypo-vitaminosis K and decreased clotting factors.

Management

1. Refer the patient to a gastroenterologist if oral ulcers are associated with bowel complaints. A gluten-free diet will reverse the symptoms.
2. Avoid aspirin or NSAIDs that inhibit platelet aggregation.
3. Assess prothrombin time before oral or periodontal surgery.

Oral Manifestation

Recurrent aphthous-like ulcerations

REGIONAL ENTERITIS (CROHN'S DISEASE)

Etiology

Unknown—immunopathologic mechanisms
Granulomatous lesions of the small bowel

Consequences for Dental Care

Bleeding diathesis
Associated oral lesions

Causes of Consequences

Inflammatory lesions of the small bowel can result in malabsorption that in turn can cause hypovitaminosis K and hypoprothrombinemia.

Management

1. Avoid aspirin and other NSAIDs that interfere with platelet adhesion.

2. Evaluate prothrombin time before oral or periodontal surgery.

Oral Manifestations

Aphthous-like ulcerations
Granulomatous nodules

ULCERATIVE COLITIS

Etiology

Unknown—stress-associated
Immunopathologic mechanisms

Consequences for Dental Care

Associated oral lesions

Cause of Consequence

Patients often have extraintestinal lesions, including ankylosing spondylitis, pyodermatitis vegetans, inflammatory liver disease, and oral lesions.

Management

Oral disease, either ulcers or pyostomatitis, generally responds well to short-term systemic steroids followed by topical steroid therapy.

Oral Manifestations

Pyostomatitis vegetans
Aphthous-like ulcerations

Hemorrhagic Diatheses and Hematologic Diseases

ANEMIA

Etiology

Iron deficiency
Intrinsic factor defect (pernicious anemia)

Folate deficiency
Internal bleeding and melana
Hemolysis and genetic defects

Consequences for Dental Care

Tiredness
Hypoxia
Sickle cell crisis
Oral carcinoma

Causes of Consequences

1. Because of decreased oxygen-carrying capacity of blood, patients are often lethargic and tire easily.
2. In sickle cell anemia (homozygote), sickle cell crises can be serious as cells sludge and can cause ischemia. Drugs that suppress the respiratory center and cause acidosis can precipitate hypoxia and crisis.

Management

1. Ensure an adequate airway throughout procedures; monitor vital signs.
2. Do not schedule lengthy appointments.
3. In patients with sickle cell anemia, avoid respiratory suppressive drugs such as narcotics and barbiturates for short-term anesthesia or sedation; avoid salicylates, which can cause acidosis.
4. Maintain inhalation oxygen nearby in case of impending cyanosis.

Oral Manifestations

Generalized pallor of mucous membranes
Bald, depapillated tongue in pernicious anemia
Oral carcinoma in Fanconi's anemia

LEUKEMIA

Etiology

Neoplasia of leukocyte blast cells, possibly oncogenic virus
    Lymphocytic
    Myelogenous

Consequences for Dental Care

Bleeding tendency
Oral infection
Delayed wound healing

Causes of Consequences

1. Leukemic cells in bone marrow crowd out megakaryocytes, leading to thrombocytopenia and bleeding.
2. Agranulocytosis can evolve because of leukemic replacement of normal myeloblasts. As a result odontogenic and periodontal infections, normally defended against by neutrophils, can progress unchecked. Normal leukocytes and erythrocytes are also required for wound repair; because they are deficient in the leukemic state, wounds repair slowly.

Management

1. Obtain complete blood count with platelet count in order to determine severity of anemia, agranulocytosis, and thrombocytopenia. Do not conduct surgery if the platelet count is below 50,000.
2. In the event of a dental or periodontal infection with a low red cell count and agranulocytosis, intravenous antibiotics may be necessary, along with eradication of the infection.
3. Do not prescribe aspirin-related analgesics for orodental pain if platelet count is low. Use acetaminophen, ibuprofen, codeine, or a combination.

Oral Manifestations

Petechial hemorrhages
Gingival enlargement

HEMOPHILIA, VON WILLEBRAND'S DISEASE, AND OTHER CLOTTING DISORDERS

Etiology

Hereditary factor deficiencies—factor VIII, von Willebrand's factor VIII, factor IX, and factor I most common
Acquired factor deficiencies
Liver disease
Malabsorption syndromes
Anticoagulant drug therapy

Consequence for Dental Care

Bleeding disorder

Cause of Consequence

Hereditary (DNA) defect for specific clotting factors leads to delayed clotting time. The intrinsic pathway (partial thromboplastin time [PTT]) is defective in factor VIII and IX deficiencies and von Willebrand's disease. The common pathway (both PTT and prothrombin time [PT]) is defective in factor I deficiency. Platelet aggregation and bleeding time are defective, along with factor VIII adhesion protein, in von Willebrand's disease.

Management

1. In documented factor deficiencies of genetic origin, all oral surgical procedures should be undertaken in the hospital, where factor administration can be prearranged.
2. For suspected factor deficiencies, assess both clotting pathways (PT, PTT) and either bleeding time or platelet aggregation.
3. In acquired factor deficiencies, obtain PT and PTT. If values are twice normal the patient should be hospitalized for oral surgical procedures.
4. Do not prescribe aspirin-related analgesics for orodental pain. Use acetaminophen, ibuprofen, codeine, or a combination.

Oral Manifestations

Ecchymosis
Oral bleeds

THROMBOCYTIC DISORDERS

Etiology

Thrombocytopenia
    Idiopathic thrombocytopenic purpura
    Leukemia
    Drug-induced
Thrombocytopathia
    Idiopathic thrombocytopathic purpura
    von Willebrand's disease
    Drug (aspirin)-induced

Consequences for Dental Care

Bleeding tendency

Causes of Consequences

1. In thrombocytopenic purpura, the decrease in platelet numbers precludes capillary plugging. In idiopathic thrombocytopenic purpura, thrombocyte autoantibodies are present; in leukemia, normal platelet production is hampered by space-occupying malignant leukocytes in the marrow. In many patients with cancer, chemotherapeutic medications will depress bone marrow.

2. In thrombocytopathia, platelets are present in adequate numbers but are defective in their ability to adhere to damaged vessel walls or they cannot aggregate to form an adequate plug in the vessel wall. Adherence- and aggregation-mediating cell surface proteins are defective in the inherited platelet disorders, and aspirin-related drugs inhibit aggregation.

Management

1. Assess the degree of defect by obtaining a platelet count and, when warranted, studies of platelet aggregation or bleeding time should be obtained. If the platelet count is below 50,000, the patient should be hospitalized and a platelet infusion arranged. If aggregation is less than 50% of normal, bleeding could be a problem.
2. Do not prescribe aspirin-related analgesics for orodental pain. Use acetaminophen, ibuprofen, codeine, or a combination.

Oral Manifestations

Mucosal petechiae

LYMPHOMA (HODGKIN'S AND NON-HODGKIN'S)

Etiology

Neoplasia of lymphocytes (some forms are associated with viruses)

Consequences for Dental Care

Possible immunocompromise due to disease or medications
Lymphoma in HIV-infected patients
Increased risk for infections
Bleeding tendency

Causes of Consequences

1. As the disease becomes disseminated, fewer functional lympho- cytes are available for circulation, so immunologic responsiveness decreases. Susceptibility to viral, fungal, and bacterial infections increases.
2. Most lymphomas are treated by combination radiation therapy and chemotherapy, which usually affects bone marrow and matu- ration of other leukocytes and platelets.
3. In intractable, nonresponsive cases, bone marrow transplantation may be considered.

Management

1. Evaluate platelet status before any oral surgical procedures.
2. Prescribe antibiotics for routine dental and periodontal infections in immunosuppressed lymphoma patients.
3. Treat candidal and herpesvirus infections with appropriate antibiotics.

Oral Manifestations

Oral lymphoma, most common on the palate or gingiva
Ulcerations secondary to chemotherapy
Candidiasis
Herpes simplex
Varicella zoster

Respiratory Diseases

CHRONIC OBSTRUCTIVE PULMONARY DISEASE

Etiology

Smoking
Bronchitis
Emphysema

Consequence for Dental Care

Inhalation anesthesia risk

Causes of Consequence

1. Bronchioles are chronically inflamed, with excessive secretions blocking airway and associated cough.
2. Alveolar air sacs in emphysema lose septae, become dilated, and do not adequately exchange gases; patient develops dyspnea.

Management

1. Shorten appointments if dyspnea is severe. Regularly and periodically allow patient to sit erect.
2. Use precautions with inhalation anesthesia because patients have defective expiration, cor pulmonale with congestive heart failure, and acidosis as a result of carbon dioxide retention.

Oral Manifestations

None

TUBERCULOSIS

Etiology

Pulmonary infection with *Mycobacterium tuberculosum*

Consequences for Dental Care

Disease transmission
Inhalation anesthesia risk

Causes of Consequences

1. In chronic active tuberculosis, organisms are found in sputum and can be disseminated around the operatory by aerosol handpieces, possibly transmitting disease to office employees or even (unlikely) other patients.
2. In active disease, there may be extensive granulomatosis and fibrosis in the lungs causing dyspnea and defective gaseous exchange, thus posing a problem during general anesthesia.
3. Miliary spread can occur to various areas in the body, including the mouth.

Management

1. Use rubber dam and rigid infection control.
2. Assess respiratory function before administration of inhalation anesthesia.
3. Perform a biopsy on any suspected oral ulcerations.

Oral Manifestation

Oral granulomatous ulcers

PNEUMOCONIOSIS

Etiology

Inhalation of particulate matter that induces pulmonary fibrosis

Consequences for Dental Care

Respiratory distress
Inhalation anesthesia risk

Causes of Consequences

1. Particulate matter from occupational exposure induces progressive fibrosis of the lung alveoli, reducing the area for gaseous

exchange. Aeration of the lungs during inhalation anesthesia or nitrous oxide analgesia may be compromised.
2. The chief agents are coal dust, silicone, asbestos, and beryllium.

Management

1. Patients with dyspnea may need to sit upright for dental procedures.
2. Pulmonary function should be ascertained before administration of inhalation anesthetics or nitrous oxide.

Oral Manifestations

None

MYCOTIC LUNG DISEASE

Etiology

Pulmonary infection with *Histoplasma, Blastomyces, Cryptococcus,* or *Coccidioides* organisms

Consequences for Dental Care

Disease transmission
Inhalation anesthesia risk

Causes of Consequences

1. In chronic active pulmonary mycosis, organisms are found in sputum and can be disseminated around the operatory by aerosol handpieces, possibly transmitting disease to office employees or even (unlikely) other patients.
2. In active disease, there may be extensive granulomatosis and fibrosis in the lungs, causing dyspnea and defective gaseous exchange, thus posing a problem for general anesthesia.
3. Miliary spread can occur to various areas in the body, including the mouth.

Management

1. Use rubber dam and rigid infection control.
2. Assess respiratory function before administration of inhalation anesthesia.
3. Perform a biopsy on any suspected oral ulcerations.

Oral Manifestation

Oral granulomatous ulcers

Endocrinopathies

DIABETES MELLITUS

Etiology

Insulin-dependent (type 1)—autoimmunity to islet cells
Non–insulin-dependent adult-onset (type 2)—decreased insulin receptors

Consequences for Dental Care

Hyperglycemic shock
Hypoglycemic shock
Delayed wound healing
Myocardial infarction risk
Oral infections

Causes of Consequences

1. Hyperglycemic shock evolves in brittle, usually type 1, diabetics who are negligent in their insulin administration or who are unaware of their disease. The ketoacidosis and hyperglycemia lead to loss of consciousness, acetone breath, dry skin and mucous membranes, tachypnea, and paralysis.
2. Hypoglycemic shock occurs in patients who take extra insulin or who fail to eat after taking insulin. The signs and symptoms include hunger, tachycardia, incoherence and confusion, paresthesias, and loss of consciousness with tonic/clonic muscular activity.
3. Microvascular disease in the periodontium affects blood flow and leukocyte immigration, predisposing to premature periodontal disease, abscesses, and delayed wound healing.
4. The vascular occlusive disease in diabetes mellitus places the patient at risk for coronary artery disease at a young age.
5. Diabetics are prone to develop oral candidiasis, periodontal abscesses, and, rarely, mucormycosis of the antrum.

Management

1. Monitor vital signs periodically throughout dental care procedures.
2. If the patient goes into hyperglycemic shock, administer insulin.
3. If the patient has a hypoglycemic episode, administer sugar.
4. Prescribe antibiotics in brittle diabetics for oral surgical procedures and for any odontogenic or periodontal acute infections.
5. Treat oral candidiasis with antifungal agents. Mucormycosis is a life-threatening infection, and the patient should be referred to an infectious disease specialist.

Oral Manifestations

Premature periodontal disease
Delayed healing after oral surgery
Candidiasis
Antral mucormycosis

DIABETES INSIPIDUS

Etiology

Neurohypophyseal lesions—inflammatory or neoplastic

Consequences for Dental Care

Oral and jaw lesions
Frequent urination

Causes of Consequences

1. Langerhans cell histiocytosis (histiocytosis X) is one cause; in it, histiocytes infiltrate various organs and tissues.
2. In the chronic disseminated form, histiocytes infiltrate the posterior pituitary, resulting in decreased output of antidiuretic hormone with resultant polyuria. Retro-orbital infiltrates may lead to exophthalmos, and osseous infiltrates are typically found in the skull and jaws.

Management

1. Langerhans cell histiocytosis is treated successfully with vinca alkaloid chemotherapy. Radiation is sometimes needed as well.
2. The jaw lesions are usually treated by local curettage; extraction of involved teeth is often required.

Oral Manifestations

Radiolucencies in the jaws, with teeth "floating in space"
Loosening of teeth

ADDISON'S DISEASE

Etiology

Idiopathic—possibly autoimmune—tuberculosis, granulomatous infection of adrenal cortex, all of which culminate in adrenal hypocorticism

Consequences for Dental Care

Low coping under stress
Hypotensive and hypoglycemic syncope

Causes of Consequences

1. Hypocorticism of the adrenal gland with a reduction in all cortico-steroids, including glucocorticoids, mineralocorticoids, and androgens.
2. Hypotension due to decreased mineralocorticoids, sodium loss, and hypovolemia.
3. Hypoglycemia secondary to decreased glucocorticoids
4. Increased output of ACTH with melanocyte-stimulating component leads to hyperpigmentation.

Management

1. Most patients with diagnosed Addison's disease are taking steroids, and the condition is therefore controlled and no particular precautions are needed.
2. In nonmedicated patients, 10 mg of prednisone daily for 3 or 4 days should be considered for dental surgery.

Oral Manifestation

Multifocal melanotic pigmentations of skin and mucosa

CUSHING'S SYNDROME

Etiology

Adrenocortical hyperplasia or adenoma
ACTH-secreting pituitary tumor
ACTH-secreting round cell malignancy

Consequences for Dental Care

Increased susceptibility to infection
Delayed wound healing
Psychologic depression

Causes of Consequences

1. Elevated steroid levels predispose to immunosuppression.
2. Collagen synthesis is inhibited by steroids.

Management

1. Prescribe antibiotics, usually penicillin-related drugs, before oral and dental surgery.
2. Monitor closely for wound repair after surgical procedures.

Oral Manifestations

Facial edema (moon facies)
Mucosal pigmentation in ACTH-secreting tumors

PREGNANCY

Etiology

We hope you know!

Consequences for Dental Care

Gingival inflammation and proliferation
Medication precautions for fetus

Causes of Consequences

1. Just as the placenta vascularizes in response to various hormonal changes, gingival tissues appear to be influenced by pregnancy-related hormonal fluctuations, perhaps because of specific hormone receptors on gingival fibroblasts and endothelial cells.
2. Embryogenesis is a delicate, controlled biologic process that can be pathologically altered by drugs and teratogens, which jeopardize fetal tissues and result in physical deformities. Radiation exposure can cause mutations in developing somatic cells. The greatest sensitivity is in the first trimester.

Management

1. Radiographs should not be taken during the first trimester except for emergency care. Abdominal shielding should be used throughout pregnancy.
2. Any medications should be evaluated thoroughly for their effects on the developing fetus and transplacental drug levels. In general, most antibiotics are safe. Prolonged narcotic analgesic therapy should not be used.
3. Because of the increase in gingivitis among some gravid women, home care may need to be more vigorous.
4. Removal of gingival reactive tumefactions often is followed by recurrence. It is therefore recommended that such lesions be treated definitively after parturition.

Oral Manifestations

Pregnancy gingivitis
Reactive proliferations of the gingiva (pyogenic granuloma)
Perioral pigmentation (malasma)

Arthritides

RHEUMATOID ARTHRITIS

Etiology

Postinfectious autoimmune inflammatory joint disease—usually subsequent to group A streptococcal infection

Consequences for Dental Care

Rheumatic heart disease may be a concomitant
Steroid and aspirin therapy can predispose to infections and bleeding
Sjögren's syndrome–associated xerostomia

Causes of Consequences

1. Poststreptococcal immunologic sequelae include cardiac valvulitis, myocarditis with arrhythmia, and glomerulonephritis.
2. Many patients are treated with steroids and NSAIDs (including aspirin), which could cause immunosuppression and platelet aggregation defects, respectively.
3. The sicca syndrome of Sjögren's syndrome includes xerostomia, xerophthalmia, and rheumatoid arthritis.

Management

1. With xerostomia present, explore for Sjögren's syndrome (SS) by biopsy of the lower lip minor salivary gland and serologic tests for antinuclear antibodies, SS, and anti-rho.
2. In heavy aspirin users, order platelet aggregation assay.
3. In Sjögren's syndrome, artificial saliva, electrostimulation of the tongue to induce salivation, pilocarpine therapy, and daily topical fluoride gels to reduce cervical caries may be necessary.

Oral Manifestations

Petechiae
Temporomandibular joint pain and crepitus
Sjögren's syndrome: xerostomia, cervical decay, parotid enlargement

GOUT

Etiology

1. Defective enzyme systems for degradation of uric acid (purine and pyrimidine [DNA] metabolites)—hereditary predisposition

Consequences for Dental Care

Medications used to treat gout may cause problems
Allopurinol
Colchicine
NSAIDs

Causes of Consequences

1. Urate crystals become deposited in joints, particularly the big toe, causing enlargement and pain. Drugs are used to increase either breakdown of purines and pyrimidines or their loss through the kidneys.
2. The chief problems for dental care involve the medications used in gout; some may increase bleeding.

Management

Evaluate for any history of prolonged bleeding or bruising. If evident, order platelet count, aggregation study, and prothrombin time.

Oral Manifestation

Rare temporomandibular joint involvement
Oral purpura

PRESENCE OF JOINT PROSTHESIS

Etiology

Arthritis
Aseptic necrosis

Consequences for Dental Care

Infection around prosthesis

Cause of Consequence

Bacteremia is a common cause. In most instances of infections in the region of a joint prosthesis, the bacteria are not of oral origin.

Management

Antibiotic coverage before dental appointments, usually with a penicillin-related drug, is recommended. Although most cases are not due to oral microorganisms, coverage is usually recommended as a precaution; however, one must be concerned with overprescribing antibiotics. Consultation with the orthopaedic surgeon is advisable to determine whether to premedicate the patient.

Oral Manifestations

None

Eye Disease

GLAUCOMA

Etiology

Increase in intraocular pressure due to inability to drain the vitreous
Wide (chronic) and narrow (acute) angle forms

Consequences for Dental Care

Some prescription drugs can increase intraocular pressure

Causes of Consequence

1. Any drug that increases intraocular pressure can cause major damage, including blindness.
2. The following drugs used in dental practice can increase intraocular pressure and should be avoided or used with care:
   a. Epinephrine
   b. Tricyclic antidepressents
   c. Steroids (systemic)
   d. Atropine, propantheline

Management

1. Refer to *Drug Information Reference* or *Physician's Desk Reference* before prescribing drugs to glaucoma patients to be certain there are no adverse effects on intraocular pressure.
2. Judicious use of anesthetic with vasoconstrictor is not a problem. Intravascular injection and administration of excessive numbers of cartridges must be avoided.
3. Use of epinephrine-soaked retraction cord is to be avoided.

Oral Manifestations

None

Clinical Laboratory Medicine: Significance of Laboratory Tests

Blood and urine samples submitted to the clinical pathology laboratory are extremely valuable adjuncts to the diagnostic process and are often used on a regular basis to monitor response to therapy. Most patients who are being monitored have copies of their laboratory test data, or such information can be obtained from the hospital chart or from the office of the attending physician. Records are not released to other practitioners without the patient's consent. A review of laboratory data is important when dental management is being considered, particularly if a bleeding diathesis is suspected.

Dental practitioners may also wish to order laboratory tests based on clinical findings at the time of examination. The most commonly ordered tests by dentists include the following:

Fasting blood glucose
Folate
Amylase
Complete blood count
Platelet count
Platelet aggregation
Prothrombin time
Partial thromboplastin time
Calcium
Alkaline phosphatase
Hepatitis B surface antigen
Hepatitis B surface antibody
Hepatitis C virus antibody
Electrolytes and blood gases
Direct immunofluorescence
Monospot
Anti-DNA
ANA
Anti-La
Anti-SSA, SSB

The more commonly ordered laboratory tests are listed here by category, in alphabetical order. Normal values are not listed since they vary from one laboratory to the next and reports typically reference the normal levels along with the patient's values. The chief disorders associated with each test are given; one should be aware, however, that other diseases not listed here may also show altered laboratory values.

BLOOD GASES AND ELECTROLYTES

Bicarbonate—elevated in alkalosis; decreased in acidosis

Calcium (Ca)—elevated in hyperparathyroidism; decreased in hypoparathyroidism

Phosphorus (P)—elevated in hypoparathyroidism and renal glomerular disease; decreased in hyperparathyroidism and renal tubular disease

Potassium (K)—increased in renal disease and adrenocortical hypofunction; decreased with certain diuretics, alkalosis, vomiting, diarrhea, nephrosis, and adrenal hypercorticism

Sodium (Na)—elevated in adrenal hypercorticism with aldosterone secretion, high intake of salt in the diet, and diabetes insipidus; decreased in alkalosis, vomiting, diarrhea, renal disease, hepatic disease, diabetes, and hypoadrenal corticism

P_{CO_2}—elevated in acidosis, decreased in alkalosis, either respiratory or metabolic

P_{O_2}—elevated in alkalosis; decreased in acidosis, either respiratory or metabolic

SERUM CHEMISTRIES

Acid phosphatase—elevated in prostatic hypertrophy and carcinoma

Adrenocorticotropic hormone (ACTH)—elevated in adrenocortical insufficiency and adrenohypercorticism of pituitary origin; decreased in hypercorticism of adrenal origin and patients taking steroids. Some nonadrenal tumors also secrete ACTH.

Albumin—decreased in liver disease, renal disease with nephrotic syndrome, and malnutrition

Aldosterone—elevated in renal disease, and adrenocortical tumors

Alkaline phosphatase—elevated in obstructive liver disease and active osteogenesis (osteitis deformans)

Amylase—elevated in parotitis and pancreatitis

Aminotransferases—elevated in active liver disease

Bilirubin, total—elevated in hepatobiliary disease and hemolytic anemias

Bilirubin, conjugated—elevated in obstructive liver disease

Calcitonin—elevated in medullary carcinoma of the thyroid and other neoplasms

Ceruloplasmin—elevated in Wilson's disease of the liver

Cholesterol—elevated in familial hyperlipoproteinemia, increased dietary fat intake, and atherosclerotic propensity; also elevated in gout, myeloma, and biliary disease.

Cortisol—elevated in hyperadrenocorticism and persons taking steroids; decreased in adrenocortical insufficiency

Creatinine—elevated in renal disease and muscle necrosis

Creatinine phosphokinase (CK), total—elevated in muscle necrosis, skeletal muscle trauma, and myocardial infarction

Creatinine phosphokinase (CK-MB)—specific for cardiac muscle; elevated in acute myocardial infarction

Cryoglobulins—elevated in autoimmune diseases, leukemia, lymphoma, myeloma, and infections

Erythropoietin (EPO)—decreased in renal disease, cis-platinum therapy

Fatty acids, free—elevated in starvation, hyperthyroidism, pheochromocytoma, and Reye's syndrome

Folate—decreased in folate-deficient anemia

Gastrin—elevated in Zollinger-Ellison syndrome and gastrin-secreting tumors

Glucose—elevated in diabetes mellitus, acute pancreatitis, hemochromatosis, and adrenal tumors; decreased in insulin-secreting tumors, renal disease, liver disease, and adrenocortical insufficiency

Glucose-6-phosphate dehydrogenase (G6PD)—deficient in a specific form of anemia

Glycosylated hemoglobin—assay of sugar bound to hemoglobin for long-term monitoring of glucose in diabetics

Hormones, sex (testosterone, estradiol, luteinizing hormone, prolactin, follicle-stimulating hormone)—assays for hormone-secreting tumors and dysfunctional disease of the menstrual cycle

Insulin—elevated in certain tumors; decreased in diabetes

Iron—increased in hemochromatosis, acute leukemia, hemolytic anemias, and pernicious anemia; decreased in iron-deficiency anemia, intestinal carcinoma with blood loss, endocarditis, nephrosis, and hypothyroidism

Lactate dehydrogenase (LDH)—elevated in tissue necrosis (particularly acute myocardial infarction); isoenzymes assayed for muscle or liver specificity

Lipase—elevated in pancreatitis

Parathormone—elevated in primary and secondary hyperparathyroidism; decreased in hypoparathyroidism

Pregnancy—test for pregnancy after 6 weeks

Protein-bound glucose—monitoring test for long-term control of blood sugar levels

Protein, total—elevated in early liver disease, chronic infection, myeloma, and cryoglobulinemia; decreased in renal disease, liver disease, malnutrition, and hypogammaglobulinemia

Renin—elevated in renovascular hypertension; secreted by some neoplasms

Thyroid hormones (T3, T4, thyroid-binding globulin)—elevated in hyperthyroidism; decreased in hypothyroidism

Thyroid-stimulating hormone (TSH)—elevated in hyperthyroidism; decreased in hypothyroidism of pituitary origin

Transferrin—elevated in iron deficiency, pregnancy, and use of contraceptives; decreased in chronic liver disease, renal disease, hemochromatosis, and hemolytic anemias

Triglycerides—elevated in familial hyperlipoproteinemias and from dietary intake, diabetes, liver disease, nephrosis, and predisposition to atherosclerosis

Urea nitrogen—elevated in renal disease (uremia)

Uric acid—elevated in gout, renal disease, and tissue necrosis; decreased in renal tubular disease and Wilson's disease

SERUM PROTEINS, ELECTROPHORESIS

Hemoglobin electrophoresis—detection of sickle cell and thalassemia hemoglobins

Immunoelectrophoresis—detection of monoclonal immunoglobulin spikes indicative of IgG, IgA, and IgM myeloma

SERUM PROTEINS, IMMUNOSEROLOGY

Alpha-fetoprotein—elevated in many neoplasms

Antinuclear antibody (ANA)—lupus erythematosus, other collagen diseases

Anti-DNA—lupus erythematosus, other collagen diseases

Anti–hepatitis A antibody (Anti–HAV Ab)—postinfection with HAV indicates immunity

Anti–hepatitis B surface antibody (Anti–HBS Ab)—postinfection or postimmunization by HBV outer envelope indicates immunity

Anti–hepatitis B core antibody (Anti–HBC Ab)—postinfection or post-immunization by HBV inner capsid protein indicates immunity

Anti–hepatitis B E antibody (Anti–HBE Ab)—immunity to infectious nuclear-associated protein of hepatitis B indicates immunity and noncarrier status

Anti–hepatitis C antibody (Anti–HCV Ab)—postinfection with HCV indicates immunity

Antimicrosomal antibody—autoimmune thyroiditis

Antimitochondrial antibody—elevated in primary biliary cirrhosis

Anti-SM, RNP—lupus erythematosus, other collagen diseases

Anti–smooth muscle antibody—autoimmune hepatitis

Anti-SSA, SBB antibody—Sjögren's syndrome

Carcinoembryonic antigen (CEA)—colon carcinoma, other neoplasms

C-reactive protein—nonspecific marker of inflammatory reactions

C1-inhibitor, quantitative—decreased in familial angioedema

Cytomegalovirus (CMV) titer—elevated in CMV infections

Complement C3/C4—decreased in familial complement deficiencies

Coxsackie A and B—herpangina, stomatitis, hand-foot-mouth disease, lymphonodular pharyngitis, and subacute thyroiditis

Epstein-Barr virus (EBV) (viral capsid antigen [VCA-IgG], EB nuclear antigen [EBNA], early antigen)—infectious mononucleosis, nasopharyngeal carcinoma, Burkitt's lymphoma)

Flourescent treponemal antibody (FTA)—syphilis

Hepatitis B surface antigen (HBSAg)—presence of viral envelope indicates current infection or carrier status

Hepatitis B E antigen (HBEAg)—presence of viral nuclear protein indicates current infection or carrier status, infectious

Herpes simplex virus (HSV)—convalesence sera elevated from herpetic infections

Human immunodeficiency virus (HIV) antibody—screening assay for HIV infection

Immune complex, PEG/C1Q—elevated in immune complex vasculitis and renal disease

Legionella **antibody**—Legionnaire's disease

Lyme antibody—Lyme disease

Prostate-specific antigen—elevated in prostatic carcinoma

Rheumatoid factor—rheumatoid arthritis, other rheumatic diseases
Rubella antibody—rubella measles
Rubeola antibody—rubeola measles
Streptolysin O antibody—streptococcal infections
Varicella Zoster (VZV) titer—elevated in chickenpox and shingles convalescence
Venereal Disease Research Laboratory (VDRL)—serologic test for syphilis
Western blot—definitive human immunodeficiency virus antibody test, indicating both latent and active infection

IMMUNOFLUORESCENCE, DIRECT

IgG or IgM and C3 pericellular—pemphigus vulgaris, pemphigus foliaceus, pyostomatitis vegetans, after penicillin therapy
IgA only, pericellular—IgA pemphigus
IgG, IgA, IgM, C3 basement membrane—linear: bullous pemphigoid, mucous membrane pemphigoid; granular: lupus erythematosus
IgA only, basement membrane—linear IgA disease
Fibrinogen basement membrane—lichen planus
IgA submucosal granular—dermatitis herpetiformis, gluten enteropathy
IgG, IgM, C3 perivascular—immune complex vasculitis, erythema multiforme
IgG, IgM, C3 nuclear—lupus erythematosus, antinuclear chronic bullous stomatitis

HEMATOLOGY AND COAGULATION

Complete Blood Count (CBC)
    Hemoglobin (Hgb)—elevated in polycythemia; decreased in anemias
    Hematocrit (Hct)—elevated in polycythemia and fluid loss; decreased in anemias
    Red cell count—elevated in polycythemia; decreased in anemias
    Red cell indices—calculated ratios from hematocrit, hemoglobin, and red cell count that compare concentration of hemoglobin and cell size (hypochromic versus hyperchromic, microcytic versus macrocytic)
    White cell count—increased with infection and leukemia; decreased in aleukemic phase of leukemia and drug-induced leukopenia
    Differential
        Blast forms in leukemia
        Myeloblasts—myelogenous
        Lymphoblasts—lymphocytic
        Neutrophilic leukocytosis—pyogenic bacteria
        Lymphocytic leukocytosis—viral and granulomatous infections
        Eosinophilia—allergy, parasitic infections

Thrombocyte count—decreased in thrombocytopenia due to cancer infiltration of marrow, various medications, consumptive coagulopathy, and platelet autoimmunity

Platelet aggregation—tests for aggregation of platelets to one another under various conditions; defects in aggregation, thrombasthenia, or thrombocytopathia may be inherited or acquired from drugs that interfere with formation of adhesion molecules

Prothrombin time (PT)—measure of the extrinsic pathway of coagulation; prolonged in chronic liver disease, hepatitis, biliary cirrhosis, warfarin therapy, steatorrhea, consumptive coagulopathy, and intrinsic factor deficiencies

Partial thromboplastin time (PTT)—measure of the intrinsic pathway of coagulation; prolonged in hemophilia, Christmas disease, Hageman factor deficiency, von Willebrand's disease, and consumptive coagulopathy

Specific factors
    Factor VIII—hemophilia
    Factor VIII–associated antigen—von Willebrand's disease
    Factor IX—Christmas disease
    Factor I—afibrinogenemia
    Factor V—factor V deficiency disease

Bleeding time—prolonged in platelet deficiency and platelet function disorders

Clotting time—prolonged in coagulation factor deficiency

Fibrin split products—disseminated intravascular coagulation

CELLULAR IMMUNOLOGY

CD4/CD8 ratio—progressive decrease in CD4 lymphocytes with time in patients infected with the human immunodeficiency virus

Kappa/lambda B cells—monoclonality for myeloma

PART

II

Medications, Drug Interactions, and Precautions

Fifty Most Frequently Prescribed Drugs

This list represents, in order of frequency, the most commonly prescribed drugs in the United States.

Generic Name	Trade Name	Class
1. amoxicillin	Amoxil	antibiotic
2. digoxin	Lanoxin	cardiostimulant
3. ranitidine	Zantac	H_2 antihistamine
4. conjugated estrogens	Premarin	sex steroid
5. alprazolam	Xanax	anxiolytic
6. hydrochlorothiazide and triamterene	Dyazide	diuretic
7. diltiazem	Cardizem	calcium channel blocker
8. thyroxine	Synthroid	hormone
9. cefaclor	Ceclor	antibiotic
10. terfenadine	Seldane	antiallergy agent
11. enalapril	Vasotec	ACE inhibitor
12. atenolol	Tenormin	beta-blocker
13. nifedipine	Procardia	calcium channel blocker
14. norethindrone and ethinyl estradiol	Ortho-Novum 7/7/7	birth control
15. captopril	Capoten	ACE inhibitor
16. naproxen	Naprosyn	NSAID
17. cimetidine	Tagamet	H_2 antihistamine
18. verapamil	Calan	calcium channel blocker
19. fluoxetine	Prozac	antidepressant
20. norethindrone and ethinyl estradiol	Ortho-Novum	birth control
21. acetaminophen and codeine	Tylenol With Codeine	analgesic
22. albuterol	Proventil Inhaler	bronchodilator
23. metoprolol	Lopressor	beta-blocker
24. amoxicillin and clavulanate	Augmentin	antibiotic
25. furosemide	Lasix	diuretic
26. diclofenac	Voltaren	NSAID
27. acetaminophen and propoxyphene	Darvocet-N 100	analgesic
28. phenytoin	Dilantin	anticonvulsant
29. theophylline	Theo-Dur	bronchodilator
30. propranolol	Inderal	beta-blocker
31. albuterol	Ventolin Inhalation Aerosol	bronchodilator
32. lovastatin	Mevacor	antilipidemic
33. triazolam	Halcion	anxiolytic
34. glyburide	Micronase	hypoglycemic
35. ciprofloxacin	Cipro	antibiotic
36. miconazole	Monistat	antifungal
37. medroxyprogesterone	Provera	sex steroid
38. amoxicillin	Generic	antibiotic
39. lovonorgestrel and ethinyl estradiol	Triphasil	sex steroid
40. potassium chloride	Micro-K	diuretic potassium replacement
41. piroxicam	Feldene	NSAID
42. acetaminophen and hydrocodone	Vicodin	analgesic

43. norgestrel and ethinyl estradiol	Lo/Ovral	sex steroid
44. hydrochlorothiazide and triamterine	Maxzide	diuretic
45. gemfibrozil	Lopid	antilipidemic
46. diazepam	Valium	anxiolytic
47. amoxicillin	Trimox	antibiotic
48. warfarin	Coumadin	anticoagulant
49. ibuprofen	Motrin	NSAID
50. glyburide	DiaBeta	hypoglycemic

ACE, angiotensin-converting enzyme; H_2 histamine; NSAID, nonsteroidal anti-inflammatory drug.

Commonly Prescribed Medications and Their Significance for Dental Practice

The most frequently prescribed drugs are benzodiazepine anxiolytics, H_2-receptor antagonists, thiazide diuretics, digitalis derivatives, beta-adrenergic antagonists, angiotensin-converting enzyme (ACE) inhibitors, penicillin and macrolide antibiotics, nonsteroidal anti-inflammatory agents (NSAIDs), and antidepressants. Other commonly prescribed drugs include other antibiotics; loop, sulfonamide, and potassium-sparing diuretics; calcium channel antagonists; central-acting, direct vasodilatory, and alpha-adrenergic antagonist anti-hypertensives; nitrates; sedatives; antipsychotics; class IA and IB antiarrhythmic agents; corticosteroids; warfarin anticoagulants; seizure-control agents; bronchodilator drugs of the beta-adrenergic agonist, anticholinergic, and theophylline classes; hypoglycemic agents; and chemotherapeutic and anticancer drugs. Many of these medications have an effect on dental management, and some interact with drugs prescribed in dentistry.

All of these pharmacologic agents can be prescribed in either generic or proprietary forms, and the lists are overwhelming. The pink section of the *Physicians' Desk Reference* is of most utility for determining the trade names of drugs. In the following sections, the medications that can affect dental care are listed according to the disease processes that they are used to treat. Only selected medications, those most often encountered, are included. The reader is referred to other drug and pharmacology texts for drugs not included in this book. Generic designations are used along with the more commonly prescribed proprietary names. Both generic and trade names can be found in alphabetical order at the end of this part; each drug is then referenced to the disease group under which it is outlined. *The drug interactions listed here are limited to those that are often prescribed in dental practice.*

EDEMA

Edema is caused by hypertension (increased blood hydrostatic pressure at the precapillary level) or hypoproteinemia from either decreased protein production as a consequence of liver disease or increased protein loss through glomeruli due to renal disease (loss of blood osmotic pressure). The drugs used to reduce edema all result in diuresis at the level of the kidney and therefore rely on some degree of renal filtration and tubular function. Many diuretics result in potassium loss and require dietary or medical supplementation of potassium salts. These drugs are commonly administered, hydrochlorothiazide being the sixth most frequently prescribed medication. Many of these drugs have an impact on dental care or produce oral side effects.

Thiazide Diuretics

GENERIC NAMES: benzoflumethiazide, benzthiazide, chlorothiazide, cyclothiazide, hydrochlorothiazide, hydroflumethiazide, methyclothiazide, polythiazide, trichlormethiazide

TRADE NAMES: Apo-Hydro, Diuril, Dyazide, Enduronyl, Esidrix, Hydro-DIURIL, Oretic, Renese

PHARMACOLOGY: Acts on distal tubule to increase excretion of water and sodium; causes potassium loss.

IMPACT ON DENTAL CARE: Xerostomia is common. Most patients taking thiazides are in congestive heart failure or are hypertensive. Appropriate precautions for these conditions must be taken. Blood dyscrasias, including thrombocytopenia and agranulocytosis, are a rare complication. Such a complication should be suspected if oral petechiae or ulcerations appear. Orthostatic hypotension may occur and can be prevented by slowly uprighting the patient from the supine position.

DRUG INTERACTIONS: Many NSAIDs decrease the hypotensive action of thiazides. Tricyclic antidepressants and barbiturates may result in a significant hypotensive episode. Steroids cause excessive potassium loss with resultant arrhythmia. Intravascularly injected anesthetic with vasoconstrictor in conjunction with potassium depletion may also predispose to arrhythmias.

Loop Diuretics

GENERIC NAMES: bumetanide, ethacrynic acid, furosemide

TRADE NAMES: Bumex, Edecrin Sodium, Lasix

PHARMACOLOGY: Decreases reabsorption of sodium and chloride at the level of the loop of Henle, resulting in diuresis

IMPACT ON DENTAL CARE: Dry mouth, although not common, may occur. Most patients on diuretics are in congestive heart failure or are hypertensive. Those being treated for liver failure may harbor a hemorrhagic diathesis. Appropriate precautions for these conditions must be taken.

DRUG INTERACTIONS: Narcotic analgesics can cause excessive hypotension. Tricyclic antidepressants and barbiturates also can cause hypotension. NSAIDs and sedatives decrease the diuretic effect. Salicylates are retained with loop diuretics. Corticoids deplete potassium with resultant arrhythmia.

Sulfonamide Diuretics

GENERIC NAMES: chlorthalidone, indapamide, metolazone, quinethazone

TRADE NAMES: Combipres, Diulo, Hygroton, Mykrox, Thalitone, Zaroxolyn

PHARMACOLOGY: Induces diuresis, with loss of sodium and chloride acting on the distal convoluted tubule

IMPACT ON DENTAL CARE: Xerostomia is common. Most patients are in congestive heart failure or are hypertensive. Appropriate precautions for these conditions must be taken. Orthostatic hypotension may occur and can be prevented by slowly uprighting the patient from the supine position.

DRUG INTERACTIONS: Steroids cause excessive potassium loss with resultant arrhythmia. Intravascularly injected anesthetic with vasoconstrictor in conjunction with potassium depletion can also predispose to arrhythmias.

Potassium-Sparing Agents

GENERIC NAMES: amiloride, spironolactone, triamterene

TRADE NAMES: Aldactone, Dyrenium, Midamor

PHARMACOLOGY: Inhibits sodium reabsorption in distal tubule with increased retention of potassium

IMPACT ON DENTAL CARE: Patients are usually in congestive failure or are hypertensive, necessitating appropriate precautions. Those with edema related to liver failure may have a bleeding tendency.

DRUG INTERACTIONS: Aspirin decreases the diuretic effect.

Carbonic Anhydrase Inhibitors

GENERIC NAME: acetazolamide

TRADE NAMES: Ak-Zol, Dazamide, Diamox

PHARMACOLOGY: Inhibits carbonic anhydrase activity in the proximal tubule, resulting in decreased reabsorption of water and specific salts

IMPACT ON DENTAL CARE: Patients often have dry mouth, dysgeusia (metallic taste), or burning mouth. Blood dyscrasias, including thrombocytopenia and agranulocytosis, can be induced by these drugs. Oral ulcerations and purpura in patients taking acetazolamide should alert one to possible drug-induced bone marrow suppression.

DRUG INTERACTIONS: Salicylates can be toxic. Ciprofloxacin can induce crystalluria. Tricyclic antidepressants can increase the antidepressant effect. Steroids can induce increased loss of potassium.

Cardiac Stimulants

GENERIC NAMES: digoxin, digitalis, digitoxin

TRADE NAMES: Crystodigin, Lanoxicaps, Lanoxin

PHARMACOLOGY: Increases stable cardiac contractility and cardiac output as a direct effect on cardiac muscle

IMPACT ON DENTAL CARE: Patients may experience headache and lethargy. Patients are usually in congestive failure or are hypertensive, neccesitating appropriate precautions.

DRUG INTERACTIONS: Erythromycin enhances digoxin absorption. Epinephrine, if injected intravascularly, can cause arrhythmia. Steroids can cause digitalis toxicity. Fluoxetine results in anxiety, confusion, and hypertension.

HYPERTENSION

Hypertension is the consequence of increased peripheral resistance or increased cardiac output. The former leads to diastolic hypertension and is the type most often treated pharmacologically because of its association with congestive heart failure and predisposition for cerebrovascular accident (stroke). Essential hypertension is insidious, often silent for years before being detected on physical examination or after the development of a medical consequence. Conversely, malignant hypertension, more common among blacks, begins at a young age, involves renal mechanisms early on, and is characterized by early-onset arteriosclerosis. The pharmacologic interventions are aimed at reducing peripheral resistance and include the use of medications that decrease vasoconstriction through a variety of mechanisms.

Angiotensin-Converting Enzyme Inhibitors

GENERIC NAMES: benazepril, captopril, enalapril, fosinopril, lisinopril, ramipril

TRADE NAMES: Altace, Apo-Capto, Capoten, Lotensin, Monopril, Prinivil, Vasotec, Zestril

PHARMACOLOGY: Prevents the conversion of angiotensin I to angiotensin II, the potent vasconstrictor and aldosterone stimulant, by angiotensin-converting enzyme (ACE)

IMPACT ON DENTAL CARE: Angioedema of the face, lips, and tongue is a complication; airway obstruction could be fatal. Bone marrow suppression could cause increased susceptibility to infection and a hemorrhagic tendency.

DRUG INTERACTIONS: NSAIDs may decrease the ACE inhibition.

Alpha-Adrenergic Antagonists

GENERIC NAMES: doxazosin, prazosin, terazosin

TRADE NAMES: Cardura, Hytrin, Minipress

PHARMACOLOGY: Blocks alpha-adrenergic receptors on vascular smooth muscle, preventing vasopressor effects of catecholamines

IMPACT ON DENTAL CARE: Dry mouth is common. When drug is first initiated, severe hypotension with syncope may occur. Orthostatic hypotension is common.

DRUG INTERACTIONS: Calcium channel blockers increase orthostatic hypotension. NSAIDs decrease effects of the antihypertensive agent.

Central-Acting Antihypertensives

GENERIC NAMES: clonidine, methyldopa

TRADE NAMES: Aldoclor, Aldomet, Aldoril, Catapres

PHARMACOLOGY: Stimulates alpha-adrenergic receptors in the brain stem, resulting in decreased sympathetic outflow to peripheral vessels, including those in the kidney; reduces blood pressure and heart rate

IMPACT ON DENTAL CARE: Some degree of sedation occurs with these medications. Xerostomia is often a complaint. Postural hypotension is a problem with methyldopa. Cervical nodes may be painful.

DRUG INTERACTIONS: Tricyclic antidepressants decrease clonidine effect and may cause a serious rise in blood pressure with methyldopa. Dapsone causes accentuated adverse erythrocyte effects.

Direct-Acting Vasodilators

GENERIC NAMES: hydralazine, minoxidil

TRADE NAMES: Apresazide, Apresoline, Loniten, Ser-Ap-Es

PHARMACOLOGY: Causes direct-acting relaxation of vascular smooth muscle, which involves calcium

IMPACT ON DENTAL CARE: Patients may experience postural hypotension.

DRUG INTERACTIONS. Steroids can increase level of absorption of minoxidil, and with hydralazine, arrhythmias may occur. Tricyclic antidepressants can cause hypotension. NSAIDs decrease the effects of hydralazine.

HYPERTENSION, ISCHEMIC HEART DISEASE

Ischemic heart disease is the result of coronary atherosclerosis, which can occur in conjunction with, or in the absence of, hypertension. Progressive coronary artery disease results in angina pectoris, particularly on exertion, and may eventually culminate in coronary occlusion, leading to arrhythmia, congestive heart failure, or cardiac arrest.

Beta-Adrenergic Antagonists

GENERIC NAMES: acebutolol, atenolol, labetalol, metoprolol, nadolol, pindolol, propranolol, timolol

TRADE NAMES: Blocadren, Cartrol, Corgard, Inderal, Lopressor, Tenormin

PHARMACOLOGY: Blocks beta-adrenergic receptors in cardiac muscle and vascular smooth muscle. Mechanisms for hypotensive effect are not well known. Beta-blockage reduces cardiac oxygen requirements, heart rate, and systolic pressure, and increases myocardial fiber length over time. Beta-blockers also have an antiarrhythmic effect, so their chief use is in the treatment of hypertension, ischemic heart disease, certain arrhythmias, and hypertrophic subaortic stenosis. They have also been used to manage pheochromocytoma-associated hypertension, hyperthyroidism, and migraine.

IMPACT ON DENTAL CARE: High stress can induce angina. Rarely, agranulocytosis occurs with increased susceptibility to infections. Lightheadedness and orthostatic hypotension may occur.

DRUG INTERACTIONS: Antihistamines are not as potent. Barbiturates can result in severe sedation. Calcium channel blockers accentuate the antihypertensive effects. Intravascular injection with vasoconstrictor could cause severe tachycardia.

Calcium Channel Blockers

GENERIC NAMES: diltiazem, felodipine, isradipine, nicardipine, nifedipine, verapamil

TRADE NAMES: Accupril, Adalat, Calan, Cardizem, Isoptin, Plendil, Procardia, Vascor

PHARMACOLOGY: Inhibits calcium influx into vascular smooth muscle and cardiac muscle, decreasing systemic peripheral resistance

IMPACT ON DENTAL CARE: Some patients have gingival fibrous hyperplasia. Dry mouth, sore throat, and nasal stuffiness also can occur. Bruising tendency may be seen.

DRUG INTERACTIONS: None of significance.

Nitrates

GENERIC NAMES: erythrityl tetranitrate, isosorbide dinitrate, nitroglycerin, pentaerythritol tetranitrate

TRADE NAMES: Cardilate, Dilatrate SR, Isotrate, Nitrocap, Nitro-Dur, Nitrogard, Nitroglyn, Nitrol, Nitronet, Nitrospan, Pentritol, Peritrate, Sorbitrate, Transderm-Nitro, Tridil

PHARMACOLOGY: Direct-acting relaxation of vascular smooth muscle, particularly coronary vessels

IMPACT ON DENTAL CARE: Emergency drug for patients with acute angina in office setting. Nitrates cause postural hypotension and tachycardia.

CARDIAC ARRHYTHMIA

Cardiac arrhythmias have many causes, ranging from those chemically induced to those that are the consequence of cardiac conduction pathway pathosis that is caused by coronary ischemia or inflammatory lesions. The agents listed here are often used in emergency situations when fibrillation or standstill is extant. They are also prescribed on a day-to-day basis for patients with conduction defects. Most of these drugs restore rhythm and increase cardiac output. Digitalis glycosides are important drugs in this group and have already been outlined under Edema.

Class IA Agents

GENERIC NAMES: disopyramide, moricizine, procainamide, quinidine

TRADE NAMES: Cardioquin, Cin-Quin, Duraquin, Ethmozine, Norpace, Novoquinidin, Procan SR, Promine, Pronestyl, Quinaglute, Quinalan, Quinate, Quinidex, Quinora

PHARMACOLOGY: Has direct effect on conduction pathways; slows conduction speed; decreases myocardial excitation; inhibits ectopic pacemaker

IMPACT ON DENTAL CARE: Patients may have xerostomia, dysgeusia, and anxiety. Procainamide and quinidine can cause bone marrow depression with neutropenia and thrombocytopenia, increasing risk for infection, ulcerative stomatitis, and bleeding.

DRUG INTERACTIONS. Barbiturates decrease antiarrhythmic effects. Anticholinergics show increased anticholinergic effects. Dapsone increases red cell damage. Intravascular epinephrine can cause serious arrhythmias. NSAIDs increase risk for bleeding.

Class IB Agents

GENERIC NAMES: mexiletine, tocainide

TRADE NAMES: Mexitil, Tonocard

PHARMACOLOGY: Inhibits inward sodium current, decreasing the rise in action potential; decreases refractory period in Purkinje fibers

IMPACT ON DENTAL CARE: Patients may have sore throat, oral ulcerations, ageusia, dysgeusia, and anxiety. Bone marrow depression with neutropenia and thrombocytopenia can occur, increasing the risk for infection, ulcerative stomatitis, and bleeding.

DRUG INTERACTIONS. Barbiturates decrease antiarrhythmic effects. Intravascular epinephrine can cause serious arrhythmias. NSAIDs increase risk for bleeding.

Class IC Agents

GENERIC NAMES: flecainide, propafenone

TRADE NAMES: Rhythmol, Tambocor

PHARMACOLOGY: Inhibits inward sodium current, decreasing the rise in action potential; prolongs refractory period in Purkinje fibers

IMPACT ON DENTAL CARE: Patients may experience ageusia, dysgeusia, xerostomia, and anxiety. Bone marrow depression with neutropenia and thrombocytopenia can occur, increasing the risk for infection, ulcerative stomatitis, and bleeding.

DRUG INTERACTIONS. Intravascular epinephrine can cause serious arrhythmias. NSAIDs increase risk for bleeding. Local anesthetics potentiate the central nervous system side effects of propafenone.

Class III Agents

GENERIC NAME: amiodarone

TRADE NAME: Cordarone

PHARMACOLOGY: Prolongs refractory period and acts noncompetitively with alpha- and beta-adrenergic inhibition

IMPACT ON DENTAL CARE: Patients may have ageusia, dysgeusia, and headache.

DRUG INTERACTIONS. Calcium channel blockers can result in heart block. Intravascular epinephrine can cause serious arrhythmias.

THROMBOEMBOLIC DISEASE

Thrombosis can occur on and in arterial and venous intimal surfaces. Arterial thrombosis is associated with high blood lipoprotein levels, and complications include ischemia, infarction, and aneurysm. Venous thrombophlebitis can eventuate in lethal pulmonary embolism. Enzyme preparations are used in acute emergency situations to clear thrombi or emboli from vessel lumina. Most of the medications prescribed on a daily basis either inhibit the synthesis of coagulation factors by interfering with vitamin K or attenuate the formation of adhesion molecules on thrombocytes. In either case, hemostasis is intentionally inhibited to prevent thrombosis. For dental surgical procedures, bleeding is the primary consideration.

Anticoagulants

GENERIC NAMES: anisindione, dicumarol, melitoxin, phenindione, warfarin

TRADE NAMES: Carfin, Coumadin, Hedulin, Miradon, Panwarfin, Sofarin

PHARMACOLOGY: Inhibits vitamin K, resulting in a deficiency of five coagulation factors and prolongation of both intrinsic and extrinsic pathways

IMPACT ON DENTAL CARE: Patients may experience hemorrhagic diathesis and prolonged or uncontrollable bleeding from oral surgical procedures.

DRUG INTERACTIONS: Acetaminophen, aspirin, fluconazole, and certain antibiotics increase bleeding. Barbiturates, tricyclic antidepressants, and fluoxetine decrease the anticoagulant effects. Benzodiazepines and antihistamines have unpredictable effects in which bleeding may be accentuated in one individual and inhibited in another.

Platelet Adhesion Inhibitors

GENERIC NAMES: dipyridamole, persantine, salicylic acid, ticlopidine

TRADE NAMES: Apo-Dipyridamole, Bufferin, Dipimol, Ecotrin, Persantin, Pyridamole, Ticlid

PHARMACOLOGY: Inhibits cyclooxygenase and phosphodiesterase pathways, resulting in a lack of platelet membrane thromboxane A_2. Ticlopidine decreases platelet adenosine diphosphate. All decrease cell-to-cell adhesion and increase the bleeding time. The platelet count remains normal unless toxic side effects occur with ticlopidine.

IMPACT ON DENTAL CARE: Patients may experience hemorrhage diathesis. Ticlopidine can induce bone marrow suppression with neutropenia and, rarely, thrombocytopenia.

DRUG INTERACTIONS: Other NSAIDs can potentiate platelet adhesion inhibition and cause a greater tendency for bleeding.

ASTHMA, DYSPNEA

Asthma is a common disease triggered by a variety of antigens or stress. Bronchospasm occurs and compromises respiratory physiology. Acute status asthmaticus can be fatal. Airway constriction is managed by bronchodilators, which are usually administered by an inhaler. When

seasonal changes cause symptoms to worsen, oral medication is often prescribed.

Xanthines

GENERIC NAMES: aminophylline, dyphilline, oxtriphylline, theophylline

TRADE NAMES: Aerolate, Asmalix, Bronkodyl, Dyflex, Lanophyllin, Marax, Neothylline, Quibron, Somophyllin, Theobid, Theo-Dur, Theolair, Theostat, Thylline

PHARMACOLOGY: Causes dilation of bronchiolar smooth muscle and increases smooth muscle cyclic adenosine monophosphate; is used mostly as an oral medication

IMPACT ON DENTAL CARE: Patients have a propensity for asthma attacks, particularly during stressful procedures.

DRUG INTERACTIONS: Ciprofloxin, clindamycin, erythromycin, and steroids increase bronchodilation. Barbiturates decrease dilation.

Adrenergic Agonists

GENERIC NAMES: adrenalin, albuterol, berotec, bitolterol, ephedrine, epinephrine, ethylnorepinephrine, fenoterol, isoetharine, isoproterenol, metaproterenol, pirbuterol, procaterol, terbutaline

TRADE NAMES: Aerolone, Alupent, AsthmaHaler, Brethine, Brontin, Bronkaid, Dey-Dose, EpiPen, Isuprel, MediHaler, Primatene, Proventil, Vapo-Iso, Ventolin

PHARMACOLOGY: Function as beta-adrenergic agonists that bind receptors and induce bronchodilation; used as tablets and as inhalers

IMPACT ON DENTAL CARE: Xerostomia is common. Patients have a propensity for asthma attacks, particularly during stressful procedures. Repeated use of inhalers can cause stomatitis, pharyngitis, and hemorrhage of mucosal bullae.

DRUG INTERACTIONS: Tricylic antidepressants can cause tachycardia and increase blood pressure. Ergot alkaloids can cause dangerous hypertension, Epinephrine increases bronchodilation.

CANCER, LYMPHOMA, LEUKEMIA

The medications used to treat cancer are toxic to dividing cells. Pharmacologically, they all inhibit the mitotic process and are therefore not restricted to dividing cancer cells but affect normal cells that typically divide regularly. The most sensitive cell populations in this regard are the hematopoietic cells of the bone marrow, gastrointestinal tract mucosal lining cells (including oral mucosa), and hair follicle germ cells. Therefore, anemia, neutropenia, immunosuppression from lym-

phopenia, thrombocytopenia, colitis, stomatitis, and hair loss are the chief complications when dosages are high. Chemotherapeutic agents are often administered in combination regimens. Some combinations are most effective for leukemias and lymphomas, whereas others are more effective for the management of solid tumors (carcinomas and sarcomas). Because most agents in this group also inhibit the immune system, some are used to treat autoimmune diseases and psoriasis.

Alkylating Agents

GENERIC NAME: cyclophosphamide

TRADE NAMES: Cytoxan, Neosar

PHARMACOLOGY: Binds DNA and inhibits mitosis

IMPACT ON DENTAL CARE: Patients are subject to bone marrow inhibition, with increased risk for infections and bleeding tendency.

DRUG INTERACTIONS: Barbiturates increase the effects of cyclophosphamide. Steroids augment immunosuppressive effects, with increased risk for infection. NSAIDs increase risk for bleeding.

GENERIC NAMES: melphalan, phenylalanine mustard (PAM, L-PAM)

TRADE NAME: Alkeran

PHARMACOLOGY: Binds to DNA and inhibits mitosis

IMPACT ON DENTAL CARE: Patients are subject to bone marrow suppression, with increased risk for infection, both candidal and odontogenic. Patients may experience hemorrhagic diathesis. Oral ulcerations indicate toxic drug levels.

DRUG INTERACTIONS: Other immunosuppressants, including steroids, compound risk for infections. NSAIDs increase risk for bleeding.

GENERIC NAME: busulfan

TRADE NAME: Myleran

PHARMACOLOGY: Binds to DNA and arrests mitosis

IMPACT ON DENTAL CARE: Patients are subject to bone marrow suppression, with increased risk of infection, both mucosal and odontogenic, and hemorrhagic tendency. Oral ulcerations indicate toxicity.

DRUG INTERACTIONS: Other immunosuppressants, including steroids, compound risk for infections. NSAIDs increase risk for bleeding.

GENERIC NAME: chlorambucil

TRADE NAME: Leukeran

PHARMACOLOGY: Binds to DNA and inhibits cell division

IMPACT ON DENTAL CARE: Patients are subject to bone marrow suppression, with increased risk of infection, both mucosal and odontogenic, and hemorrhagic tendency. Oral ulcerations indicate toxicity.

DRUG INTERACTIONS: Immunosuppressant drugs (such as steroids) potentiate the risk for infection. NSAIDs increase risk for bleeding.

Antimetabolites

GENERIC NAME: methotrexate

TRADE NAMES: Folex, Mexate-AQ, Rheumatex

PHARMACOLOGY: Inhibits dihydrofolic acid reductase and formation of an essential metabolite for purine synthesis

IMPACT ON DENTAL CARE: Patients are subject to bone marrow inhibition, with increased risk for infections and bleeding tendency. Orthostatic hypotension is also an effect.

DRUG INTERACTIONS: NSAIDs, aspirin, and tetracyclines increase methotrexate toxicity and bone marrow suppression. NSAIDs increase risk for bleeding.

GENERIC NAME: mercaptopurine

TRADE NAMES: 6-MP, Purinethol

PHARMACOLOGY: Functions as a false nucleotide, preventing mitosis by inhibiting normal purine synthesis.

IMPACT ON DENTAL CARE: Patients are subject to bone marrow suppression, with increased risk of infection, both mucosal and odontogenic, and hemorrhagic tendency. Oral ulcerations indicate toxicity.

DRUG INTERACTIONS: With acetaminophen, liver toxicity is common. Other immunosuppressants, including steroids, increase risk for infections. NSAIDs increase risk for bleeding.

GENERIC NAME: hydroxyurea

TRADE NAME: Hydrea

PHARMACOLOGY: Inhibits DNA synthesis without affecting RNA or protein synthesis; exact mechanism unknown

IMPACT ON DENTAL CARE: Effects of hydroxyurea are usually minor compared with other anticancer medications. It may cause stomatitis.

DRUG INTERACTIONS: Other immunosuppressants may predispose to oral infections.

GENERIC NAME: cytarabine

TRADE NAME: Cytosar-U

PHARMACOLOGY: Inhibits DNA polymerase, arresting mitosis

IMPACT ON DENTAL CARE: Patients are subject to marrow suppression, with increased susceptibility to infections, both mucosal and dental, and hemorrhagic tendency.

DRUG INTERACTIONS: Other immunosuppressants may predispose to oral infections. NSAIDs increase risk for bleeding.

AUTOIMMUNE/COLLAGEN DISEASE, ORGAN TRANSPLANTATION

The immunosuppressive medications in this category are prescribed for patients with overactive immune systems and include drugs that inhibit both B- and T-lymphocyte functions. The primary short-term uses are for allergic reactions; long-term therapy is used to treat autoimmune and collagen diseases as well as to allow acceptance of transplanted organs or to prevent graft-verus-host disease in patients with bone marrow transplants and peripheral blood stem cell infusions. Prolonged immunosuppression predisposes to infections of skin and mucous membranes. Ordinary dental and periodontal infections can become more severe.

Cortical Steroids

GENERIC NAMES: cortisone, dexamethasone, methylprednisolone, prednisone

TRADE NAMES: Dalalone, Decadron, Delta-Cortef, Depo-Medrol, Dexasone, Dexone, Duralone, Hexadrol, Kenalog, Medralone, Medrol, Solu-Medrol

PHARMACOLOGY: The actions of corticoids are protean, with anti-inflammatory effects on leukocytes, endothelial cells, and fibroblasts. Antibody synthesis is attenuated, neutrophil lysosomal and other antimicrobial proteins are inhibited, and lymphocyte interactions are inhibited.

IMPACT ON DENTAL CARE: High levels predispose to infections, particularly candidiasis. Odontogenic and periodontal infections may become more severe or prolonged. Antibiotic and antifungal medications may be indicated.

DRUG INTERACTIONS: NSAIDs aggravate peptic ulcer. Barbiturates decrease steroid effects.

Antimetabolites

Some antimetabolites are used to treat rheumatoid arthritis, pemphigus vulgaris, and psoriasis (chlorambucil, cyclophosphamide, mercaptopurine). Refer to Chemotherapeutic Agents.

Nonsteroidal Immunosuppressants

GENERIC NAMES: azathioprine, cyclosporine

TRADE NAMES: Imuran, Sandimmune

PHARMACOLOGY: Has complex effects on B and T lymphocytes, with inhibition of antibody synthesis, immunoregulatory mechanisms, and cytokine release

IMPACT ON DENTAL CARE: Immunosuppressants predispose patients to candidiasis and may accentuate bacterial infections of pulpal, periapical, and periodontal origin. Cyclosporine causes gingival enlargement in some patients.

DRUG INTERACTIONS: Chronic use of other immunosuppressants increases susceptibility to infection and predisposes patients to development of cancer. Erythromycin increases effect of cyclosporine. Vancomycin, ketoconazole, dapsone, and NSAIDs increase risk for renal toxicity.

SEIZURES

Epilepsy is the most common form of seizure disorder and is subdivided into petit mal and grand mal, according to severity. Hydantoin is the primary anticonvulsant used to treat grand mal seizures, whereas succinimides and diones are more often used for absence or petit mal epilepsy. Other drugs that can be used alone or in combination with hydantoin are barbiturates and benzodiazepines, listed here under Anxiety. Seizures can also occur as a consequence of organic brain lesions such as tumor or stroke. Episodic trigeminal neuralgia is treated with antiseizure drugs, usually carbamazepine.

Hydantoins

GENERIC NAMES: ethotoin, mephenytoin, phenytoin

TRADE NAMES: Dilantin, Diphenylan, Mesantoin, Peganone

PHARMACOLOGY: Stabilizes threshold for excitability in motor cortex neurons by affecting membrane sodium gradients

IMPACT ON DENTAL CARE: There is a tendency for anxiety to precipitate seizures even when the patient is taking medication. Gingival hyperplasia associated with hydantoins is related to dental plaque irritants. Although rare, bone marrow suppression can occur, with increased bleeding and susceptibility for infections. Hydantoins can also induce a lupus-like syndrome.

DRUG INTERACTIONS: Tricyclic antidepressants and fluconazole potentiate seizure suppression. Barbiturates increase sedation and alter seizure patterns. Corticosteroids are less effective as immunosuppressive agents.

Dione Anticonvulsants

GENERIC NAMES: paramethadione, trimethadione

TRADE NAMES: Paradione, Tridione

PHARMACOLOGY: Has sedative effects effective in petit mal but not grand mal epilepsy

IMPACT ON DENTAL CARE: Severe bone marrow depression can occur, with neutropenia and thrombocytopenia, resulting in ulcerative stomatitis, bleeding tendency, and increased risk for oral and dental infections.

DRUG INTERACTIONS: Antidepressants increase risk for seizures. Fluoxetine can increase sedation. Other sedatives and anxiolytics cause severe sedation.

Succinimides

GENERIC NAMES: Ethosuximide, methsuximide, phensuximide

TRADE NAMES: Celontin, Milontin, Zarontin

PHARMACOLOGY: Suppresses paroxysmal losses of consciousness associated with absence seizures

IMPACT ON DENTAL CARE: Succinimides have minimal effects besides drowsiness and headache

DRUG INTERACTIONS: Tricyclic antidepressants can provoke seizures.

Other

GENERIC NAME: Carbamazepine

TRADE NAMES: Epitol, Tegretol

PHARMACOLOGY: Reduces polysynaptic responses and blocks post-tetanic potentiation; depresses thalamic and bulbar synapses

IMPACT ON DENTAL CARE: Carbamazepine is used in the treatment of trigeminal neuralgia. It causes bone marrow depression and neutropenia at higher dosages, with increased risk for infection.

DRUG INTERACTIONS: Tricyclic antidepressants and fluoxetine can cause confusion and psychosis. Steroids are less effective when given with carbamazepine. Erythromycins suppress analgesic effects.

DEPRESSION

The psychologic disorders of affect are common, and antidepressant medications are among the most commonly prescribed drugs. The tricyclic and tetracyclic antidepressants tend to cause dry mouth, and many drug interactions occur. Many new non–tricyclic antidepressant medi-

cations are being released and used extensively. Most of these newer medications do not have anticholinergic effects and are not as prone to cause awakening drowsiness.

Tricyclic Antidepressants

GENERIC NAMES: amitriptyline, amoxapine, clomipramine, desipramine, doxepin, imipramine, nortriptyline, protriptyline, trimipramine

TRADE NAMES: Adapin, Anafranil, Aventyl, Elavil, Norpramin, Novo-pramine, Sinequan, Tofranil

PHARMACOLOGY: Elevates mood; prevents reuptake of norepinephrine and serotonin at adrenergic and serotonergic synapses

IMPACT ON DENTAL CARE: Xerostomia is common.

DRUG INTERACTIONS: Antihistamines, barbiturates, benzodiazepines, and narcotic analgesics increase sedation. Antihistaminic effects are increased, and barbiturates decrease the antidepressant effects.

Others

GENERIC NAME: trazodone

TRADE NAME: Desyrel

PHARMACOLOGY: Elevates mood; prevents reuptake of serotonin

IMPACT ON DENTAL CARE: Xerostomia is common.

DRUG INTERACTIONS: Excess sedation can occur with tricyclic antidepressants, antihistamines, barbiturates, benzodiazepines, and narcotics. Barbiturates cause hypotension.

GENERIC NAMES: fluoxetine, paroxetine

TRADE NAMES: Paxil, Prozac

PHARMACOLOGY: Elevates mood; prevents reuptake of serotonin

IMPACT ON DENTAL CARE: Dry mouth is rarely encountered. Oral ulcers may occur.

DRUG INTERACTIONS: Excess sedation can occur with tricyclic antidepressants, antihistamines, barbiturates, benzodiazepines, and narcotics.

ANXIETY

High-stress life experiences sometimes create anxiety states that can incapacitate people. Some anxiety conditions are reactive and resolve with time and psychotherapy or counseling; others are chronic and can persist for years. Short-term treatment lasting only a few days may be prescribed for phobias. Most anxiolytic medications are addictive, as are sedative / hypnotic drugs. Many of these anxiolytics are also useful in the prevention of seizure disorders. Care must be taken when prescribing medications that accentuate the effects of this class of drugs, since severe sedation can occur.

Benzodiazepines

GENERIC NAMES: alprazolam, chlorazepate, chlordiazepoxide, clonazepam, diazepam, flurazepam, lorazepam, midazolam, oxazepam, prazepam, temazepam, triazolam

TRADE NAMES: Alzapam, Ativan, Centrax, Dalmane, Durapam, Klonopin, Librium, Mogadon, Paxipam, ProSom, Serax, Tranxene, Valium, Xanax, Zetran

PHARMACOLOGY: Acts on limbic system, thalamus, and hypothalamus to produce a calming effect; appears to inhibit presynaptic transmission and is associated with elevated gamma amino butyric acid

IMPACT ON DENTAL CARE: Benzodiazepines may benefit phobic patients. Drug interactions are common, and these drugs are potentially addictive.

DRUG INTERACTIONS: Antihistamines, antidepressants, erythromycin, ketoconazole, narcotics, other anxiolytics, and barbiturates all increase the level of sedation.

Barbiturates

GENERIC NAMES: amobarbital, aprobarbital, mephobarbital, metharbital, pentobarbital, phenobarbital, secobarbital, talbutal

TRADE NAMES: Amytal, Butisol, Gemonil, Mebaral, Nembutal, Novopentobarb, Seconal, Solfoton, Tuinal; combination formulations with belladonna alkaloids: Anaspaz, Antrocol, Barbidonna, Bellergal, Butibel, Donnatal, Relaxadon, Spasmolin, Spasmophen

PHARMACOLOGY: Causes depression of sensory cortex function, motor function, and cerebellar function by delaying synaptic recovery with enhancement of gamma amino butyric acid; has anesthetic effects at high doses

IMPACT ON DENTAL CARE: Barbiturates cause drowsiness, which may be of benefit for phobic patients. Many drug interactions induce respiratory depression.

DRUG INTERACTIONS: Nitrous oxide induction phase may induce severe respiratory depression. Antidepressants, antihistamines, benzodiazepines, and narcotics all cause marked sedation and predispose to respiratory arrest. Aspirin and carbamazepine effects are decreased.

PSYCHOSIS

Many psychoses are inherited and involve biochemical defects in neuro-transmitter mechanisms. Although psychotherapy continues to be a major form of therapeutic intervention, medications can also be used to influence both affective disorders and major psychotic illnesses, including schizophrenia, paranoia, and bipolar disorders. Most of these drugs act directly on the central nervous system and have effects on motor function and consciousness. Their primary dental impact involves drug interactions.

Phenothiazines

GENERIC NAMES: acetophenazine, chlorpromazine, fluphenazine, mesoridazine, methotrimeprazine, pericyazine, perphenazine, pipotiazine, prochlorperazine, promazine, thiopropazate, thioproperazine, thioridazine, trifluoperazine, triflupromazine

TRADE NAMES: Compazine, Mellaril, Permitil, Prolixin, Prozine-50, Serentil, Stelazine, Suprazine, Thorazine, Tindal, Trilafon, Vesprin

PHARMACOLOGY: Acts at all levels of the central nervous system, inducing a neuroleptic sedative effect. Extrapyramidal excitation is a significant side effect, and autonomic neurotransmitters are blocked with atropine-like anticholinergic effects, as well as antiadrenergic effects.

IMPACT ON DENTAL CARE: Extrapyramidal effects may result in lingual, facial, and masticatory muscle spasms. Xerostomia and postural hypotension are commonly seen. Rare instances of bone marrow depression with neutropenia and ulcerative stomatitis occur.

DRUG INTERACTIONS: Anticholinergics have an increased effect when taken concurrently with phenothiazines. Tricyclic antidepressants potentiate the effects of phenothiazines. Antihistamine effects are increased. Anxiolytic drugs and barbiturates cause increased sedation, as do narcotic analgesics.

Lithium

GENERIC NAME: lithium salts

TRADE NAMES: Cibalith-S, Eskalith, Lithane, Lithobid, Lithonate, Lithotabs

PHARMACOLOGY: Prevents manic behavior; mechanism not known, but involves alteration in neuronal sodium transport that affects intracellular catecholamines

IMPACT ON DENTAL CARE: Dry mouth is sometimes encountered.

DRUG INTERACTIONS: NSAIDs and carbamazepine increase levels or effects of lithium. Metronidazole can cause lithium toxicity. Excessive sedation may be seen with antihistamines and anxiolytics. Benzodiazepines can result in hypothermia. Muscle relaxants have increased effects.

Butyrophenones

GENERIC NAME: haloperidol

TRADE NAME: Haldol

PHARMACOLOGY: Has antipsychotic, sedative effects

IMPACT ON DENTAL CARE: Butyrophenones cause xerostomia and have extrapyramidal effects, with spastic tongue, jaw, and facial movements.

DRUG INTERACTIONS: Sedative and hypotensive effects are increased with barbiturates, benzodiazepines, antihistamines, narcotic analgesics, and tricyclic antidepressants. Anticoagulant effects of phenindione are decreased.

Rauwolfia Alkaloids

GENERIC NAMES: alseroxylon, deserpidine, rauwolfia serpentina, reserpine

TRADE NAMES: Demi-Regroton, Harmonyl, Rauval, Rauzide, Regroton, Serpasil

PHARMACOLOGY: Inhibits epinephrine uptake into storage granules; has direct sedative central nervous system effect

IMPACT ON DENTAL CARE: Xerostomia is common.

DRUG INTERACTIONS: Antihistamines have increased effect; aspirin has decreased effect. Fluoxetine increases depression.

PAIN

Both narcotic and nonnarcotic analgesics are used to treat pain, and many are formulated with other drugs that potentiate the others' analgesic effects. These drugs are, of course, commonly prescribed in dentistry. Nevertheless, many patients seeking dental care may be taking pain medications for nondental acute or chronic pain. These drugs will not be reviewed here since they are detailed in Part VI.

ENDOCRINOPATHY, CONTRACEPTION

Hormonal diseases occur when either hyposecretion or hypersecretion from an endocrine organ occurs. Deficiencies are the consequence of inflammatory lesions that destroy secretory cells, whereas hypersecre-

tion occurs as a result of endocrine gland hyperplasias or neoplasms. Many hormonal therapeutic interventions are done for diabetes, hypothyroidism, osteoporosis in women, dysmenorrhea, and birth control.

Hypoglycemics

GENERIC NAMES: acetohexamide, chlorpropamide, glipizide, glyburide, tolazamide, tolbutamide

TRADE NAMES: DiaBeta, Diabinese, Glucamide, Glucotrol, Micronase, Oramide, Orinase, Tolamide, Tolinase

PHARMACOLOGY: Activates beta cells to increase insulin output

IMPACT ON DENTAL CARE: Hypoglycemics may cause erythema multiforme–like reactions in the mouth.

DRUG INTERACTIONS: Aspirin and fluconazole lower glucose to a greater degree. Steroids raise blood sugar even in the presence of hypoglycemic agents. Dapsone increases red cell damage.

Insulins

GENERIC NAMES: animal insulins, protamine zinc iletin, recombinant human insulins

TRADE NAMES: Humulin, Insulatard, Lente, Lente Iletin, Mixtard, Novolin, NPH, Semilente, Ultralente, Velosulin

PHARMACOLOGY: Replaces missing insulin in diabetic patients. It is taken by injection or by insulin pump, and glucose levels and glycosylated hemoglobin levels can be monitored. Chemical modifications of the insulin preparations vary the duration of activity.

IMPACT ON DENTAL CARE: Brittleness is common among insulin-dependent diabetics. Hyperglycemic and hypoglycemic shock must be considered and precautions taken. Complications of diabetes occur in the oral cavity, but insulin has no adverse effects on orofacial tissues. Medical records should be reviewed before treatment.

DRUG INTERACTIONS: Epinephrine and steroids increase blood sugar. Nicotine cessation interventions increase the effects of insulin, as do salicylates, sulfa antibiotics, and tetracyclines, thereby potentiating hypoglycemia.

Thyroxine

GENERIC NAMES: levothyroxin, thyroxine (T_4)

TRADE NAMES: Levothroid, Levoxine, Synthroid

PHARMACOLOGY: Acts as a substitute for thyroid hormone in patients with hypothyroidism

IMPACT ON DENTAL CARE: Unless dosage is too high, there is no significant impact on dental care other than potential for drug interactions. Overdose will accentuate nervousness and dental phobias.

DRUG INTERACTIONS: Tricyclic antidepressant effects are increased. Aspirin increases effects of thyroxine. Barbiturate effects are attenuated. Intravascular epinephrine may cause arrhythmia. Steroid effects are decreased.

Oral Contraceptives

GENERIC NAMES: ethynodiol and estradiol, levonorgestrel and estradiol, norethindrone and estradiol, norethindrone and mestranol, norethynodrel and mestranol, norgestrel and estradiol

TRADE NAMES: Demulen, Enovid, Genora, Loestrin, Lo/Ovral, Modicon, Norcept-E, Nordette, Norlestrin, Ortho-Novum, Ovcon, Ovulen

PHARMACOLOGY: Interferes with fertility by inhibiting release of follicle-stimulating hormone and luteinizing hormone, preventing ovulation

IMPACT ON DENTAL CARE: Malasma is a rare complication. Facial hair may increase.

DRUG INTERACTIONS: Ampicillin, antihistamines, barbiturates, and tetracycline decrease contraceptive effects and may result in unwanted pregnancy. Tricyclic antidepressants may have adverse effects.

Estrogens

GENERIC NAMES: chlorotrianisene, conjugated estrogens, diethylstilbestrol, esterified estrogens, estrone, estropipate, ethinyl estradiol, quinestrol

TRADE NAMES: Brevicon, Delestrogen, Demulen, Depo-Estradiol, Dura-Estrin, Duragen, Estinyl, Estrace, Estronol, Feminone, Gynogen, Loestrin, Modicon, Norinyl, Norlestrin, Ogen, Ovcon, Premarin, Stilphostrol, Tace, Tri-Norinyl, Valergen

PHARMACOLOGY: Acts as a replacement for physiologic estrogen after menopause and in instances of low estrogen and cycle irregularities; also inhibits osteoporosis

IMPACT ON DENTAL CARE: Estrogen has no significant effects beyond occasional malasma.

DRUG INTERACTIONS: Tricyclic antidepressants may become more toxic. Carbamazepine and barbiturates can decrease estrogen effects.

Alphabetical Listing Referenced to Disease Processes

Accupril—hypertension, ischemic heart disease
acebutolol—hypertension, ischemic heart disease
acetazolamide—edema
acetohexamide—endocrinopathy, contraception
acetophenazine—psychosis
Adalat—hypertension, ischemic heart disease
Adapin—depression
adrenalin—asthma
Aerolate—asthma
Aerolone—asthma
Ak-Zol—edema
albuterol—asthma
Aldactone—edema
Aldoclor—hypertension
Aldomet—hypertension
Aldoril—hypertension
Alkeran—cancer, lymphoma, leukemia
alprazolam—anxiety
alseroxylon—psychosis
Altace—hypertension
Alupent—asthma
Alzapam—anxiety
amiloride—edema
aminophylline—asthma
amiodarone—cardiac arrhythmia
amitriptyline—depression
amobarbital—anxiety
amoxapine—depression
Amytal—anxiety
Anafranil—depression
Anaspaz—anxiety
anisindione—thromboembolic disease
Antrocol—anxiety
apo benzodiazepines, generics—anxiety
apo-phenothiazines, generics—psychosis
Apresazide—hypertension
Apresoline—hypertension
aprobarbital—anxiety
Asmalix—asthma
aspirin—thromboembolic disease
AsthmaHaler—asthma
atenolol—hypertension, ischemic heart disease
Ativan—anxiety
Atropine—anxiety

Aventyl—depression
azathioprine—autoimmune/collagen disease, organ transplantation

Barbidonna—anxiety
Bellergal-S—anxiety
benazepril—hypertension
benzoflumethiazide—edema
benzthiazide—edema
bepridil—hypertension, ischemic heart disease
berotec—asthma
bitolterol—asthma
Blocadren—hypertension, ischemic heart disease
Brethine—asthma
Brevicon—endocrinopathy, contraception
Bronkaid—asthma
Bronkodyl—asthma
Brontin—asthma
Bufferin—thromboembolic disease
bumetadine—edema
Bumex—edema
busulfan—cancer, lymphoma, leukemia
butabarbital—anxiety
Butibel—anxiety
Butisol—anxiety

Calan—hypertension, ischemic heart disease
Capoten—hypertension
carbamazepine—seizures
Cardilate—hypertension, ischemic heart disease
Cardioquin—cardiac arrhythmia
Cardizem—hypertension, ischemic heart disease
Cardura—hypertension
Carfin—thromboembolic disease
carteolol—hypertension, ischemic heart disease
Cartrol—hypertension, ischemic heart disease
Catapres—hypertension
Celontin—seizures
Centrax—anxiety
chlorambucil—cancer, lymphoma, leukemia
chlorazepate—anxiety
chlordiazepoxide—anxiety
chlorothiazide—edema
chlorotrianisene—endocrinopathy, contraception
chlorpromazine—psychosis
chlorpropamide—endocrinopathy, contraception
chlorthalidone—edema

Cibalith-S—psychosis
Cin-Quin—cardiac arrhythmia
clomipramine—depression
clonazepam—anxiety
clonidine—hypertension
clorazepate—anxiety
Combipres—edema
Compazine—psychosis
conjugated estrogens—endocrinopathy, contraception
Cordarone—cardiac arrhythmia
Corgard—hypertension, ischemic heart disease
cortisone—autoimmune/collagen disease, organ transplantation
Coumadin—thromboembolic disease
Crystodigin—edema
cyclophosphamide—cancer, lymphoma, leukemia
cyclosporine—autoimmune/collagen disease, organ transplantation
cyclothiazide—edema
cytarabine—cancer, lymphoma, leukemia
Cytosar-U—cancer, lymphoma, leukemia
Cytoxan—cancer, lymphoma, leukemia

Dalalone—autoimmune/collagen disease, organ transplantation
Dalmane—anxiety
Dazamide—edema
Decadrone—autoimmune/collagen disease, organ transplantation
Delestrogen—endocrinopathy, contraception
Delta-Cortef—autoimmune/collagen disease, organ transplantation
Demi-Regroton—psychosis
Demulen—endocrinopathy, contraception
Depogen—endocrinopathy contraception
Depo-Estradiol—endocrinopathy, contraception
Depo-Medrol—autoimmune/collagen disease, organ transplantation
deserpidine—psychosis
desipramine—depression
Desyrel—depression
dexasone—autoimmune/collagen disease, organ transplantation
dexamethasone—autoimmune/collagen disease, organ transplantation
Dexone—autoimmune/collagen disease, organ transplantation
Dey-Dose—asthma
DiaBeta—endocrinopathy contraception
Diabinese—endocrinopathy, contraception
Diamox—edema
diazepam—anxiety
dicumarol—thromboembolic disease
diethylstilbestrol—endocrinopathy, contraception

digitalis—edema
digitoxin—edema
digoxin—edema
Dilatrate SR—hypertension, ischemic heart disease
Dilantin—seizures
diltiazem—hypertension, ischemic heart disease
Diphenylan—seizures
Dipimol—thromboembolic disease
dipyridamole—thromboembolic disease
disopyramide—cardiac arrhythmia
Diudhlor H—edema
Diulo—edema
Diuril—edema
Donnatal—anxiety
doxazosin—hypertension
doxepin—depression
Dura-Estrin—endocrinopathy, contraception
Duragen—endocrinopathy, contraception
Duralone—autoimmune/collagen disease, organ transplantation
Durapam—anxiety
Duraquin—cardiac arrhythmia
Dyazide—edema
Dyflex—asthma
dyphylline—asthma
Dyrenium—edema

Ecotrin—thromboembolic disease
Edecrin Sodium—edema
Elavil—depression
Enalapril—hypertension
Enduronyl—edema
Enovid—endocrinopathy, contraception
ephedrine—asthma
epinephrine—asthma
EpiPen—asthma
Epitol—seizures
erythrityl tetranitrate—hypertension, ischemic heart disease
Esidrix—edema
Eskalith—psychosis
esterified estrogens—endocrinopathy, contraception
Estinyl—endocrinopathy, contraception
Estrace—endocrinopathy, contraception
estrone—endocrinopathy, contraception
Estronol—endocrinopathy, contraception
estropipate—endocrinopathy, contraception
ethacrynic acid—edema
ethinyl estradiol—endocrinopathy, contraception

Ethmozine—cardiac arrhythmia
ethosuximide—seizures
ethotoin—seizures
ethylnorepinephrine—asthma
ethynodiol and estradiol—endocrinopathy, contraception

felodipine—hypertension, ischemic heart disease
Feminone—endocrinopathy, contraception
fenoterol—asthma
flecainide—cardiac arrhythmia
fluoxetine—depression
fluphenazine—psychosis
flurazepam—anxiety
Folex—cancer, lymphoma, leukemia
fosinopril—hypertension

Gemonil—anxiety
Genora—endocrinopathy, contraception
glipizide—endocrinopathy, contraception
Glucamide—endocrinopathy, contraception
Glucotrol—endocrinopathy, contraception
glyburide—endocrinopathy, contraception
Gynogen—endocrinopathy, contraception

halazepam—anxiety
Haldol—psychosis
haloperidol—psychosis
Harmonyl—psychosis
Hedulin—thromboembolic disease
Hexadrol—autoimmune/collagen disease, organ transplantation
Humulin—endocrinopathy, contraception
hydralazine—hypertension
Hydrea—cancer, lymphoma, leukemia
hydrochlorothiazide—edema
HydroDIURIL—edema
hydroflumethiazide—edema
hydroxyurea—cancer, lymphoma, leukemia
Hygroton—edema
Hytrin—hypertension

imipramine—depression
Imuran—autoimmune/collagen disease, organ transplantation
indapamide—edema
Inderal—hypertension, ischemic heart disease

Insulatard—endocrinopathy, contraception
insulin—endocrinopathy, contraception
isoetharine—asthma
isoproterenol—asthma
Isoptin—hypertension, ischemic heart disease
isosorbide dinitrate—hypertension, ischemic heart disease
Isotrate—hypertension, ischemic heart disease
isradipine—hypertension, ischemic heart disease
Isuprel—asthma

Kenalog—autoimmune/collagen disease, organ transplantation
Klonopin—anxiety

labetalol—hypertension, ischemic heart disease
Lanophyllin—asthma
Lanoxicaps—edema
Lanoxin—edema
Lente Iletin—endocrinopathy, contraception
Lente insulin—endocrinopathy, contraception
Leukeran—cancer, lymphoma, leukemia
levonorgestrel and estradiol—endocrinopathy, contraception
Levothroid—endocrinopathy, contraception
levothyroxine—endocrinopathy, contraception
Levoxine—endocrinopathy, contraception
Librium—anxiety
lisinopril—hypertension
Lithane—psychosis
Lithobid—psychosis
Lithonate—psychosis
Lithotabs—psychosis
Loestrin—endocrinopathy, contraception
Loniten—hypertension
Lo/Ovral—endocrinopathy, contraception
Lopressor—hypertension, ischemic heart disease
lorazepam—anxiety
Lotensin—hypertension

Marax—asthma
Mebaral—anxiety
MediHaler—asthma
Medralone—autoimmune/collagen disease, organ transplantation
Medrol—autoimmune/collagen disease, organ transplantation
melitoxin—thromboembolic disease
Mellaril—psychosis
melphalan—cancer, lymphoma, leukemia

mephenytoin—seizures
mephobarbital—anxiety
mercaptopurine—cancer, lymphoma, leukemia
Mesantoin—seizures
mesoridazine—psychosis
metaproterenol—asthma
metharbital—anxiety
methotrexate—cancer, lymphoma, leukemia
methotrimeprazine—psychosis
methsuximide—seizures
methyclothiazide—edema
methyldopa—hypertension
methylprednisolone—autoimmune/collagen disease, organ trans-
    plantation
metolazone—edema
metoprolol—hypertension, ischemic heart disease
Mexate-AQ—cancer, lymphoma, leukemia
mexiletine—cardiac arrhythmia
Mexitil—cardiac arrhythmia
Micronase—antidiabetic
Midamor—edema
midazolam—anxiety
Milontin—seizures
Minipress—hypertension
minoxidil—hypertension
Miradon—thromboembolic disease
Mixtard—endocrinopathy, contraception
Modicon—endocrinopathy, contraception
Mogadon—anxiety
Monopril—hypertension
moricizine—cardiac arrhythmia
6-MP—cancer, lymphoma, leukemia
Mykrox—edema
Myleran—cancer, lymphoma, leukemia

nadolol—hypertension, ischemic heart disease
Nembutal—anxiety
Neosar—cancer, lymphoma, leukemia
Neothylline—asthma
nicardipine—hypertension, ischemic heart disease
nifedipine—hypertension, ischemic heart disease
Nitrocap—hypertension, ischemic heart disease
Nitro-Dur—hypertension, ischemic heart disease
Nitrogard—hypertension, ischemic heart disease
nitroglycerin—hypertension, ischemic heart disease
Nitroglyn—hypertension, ischemic heart disease
Nitrol—hypertension, ischemic heart disease

Nitronet—hypertension, ischemic heart disease
Nitrospan—hypertension, ischemic heart disease
Norcept-E—endocrinopathy, contraception
Nordette—endocrinopathy, contraception
norethindrone and estradiol—endocrinopathy, contraception
norethynodrel and mestranol—endocrinopathy, contraception
norgestrel and estradiol—endocrinopathy, contraception
Norlestrin—endocrinopathy, contraception
Norpace—cardiac arrhythmia
Norpramin—depression
nortriptyline—depression
Novolin—endocrinopathy, contraception
NPH—endocrinopathy, contraception

Ogen—endocrinopathy, contraception
Oramide—endocrinopathy, contraception
Oretic—edema
Orinase—endocrinopathy, contraception
Ortho-Novum—endocrinopathy, contraception
Ovcon—endocrinopathy, contraception
Ovulen—endocrinopathy, contraception
oxazepam—anxiety
oxtriphylline—asthma

Panwarfin—thromboembolic disease
Paradione—seizures
paramethadione—seizures
paroxetin—depression
Paxil—depression
Paxipam—anxiety
Peganone—seizures
pentaerythritol tetranitrate—hypertension, ischemic heart disease
pentobarbital—anxiety
Pentritol—hypertension, ischemic heart disease
pericyazine—psychosis
Peritrate—hypertension, ischemic heart disease
Permitil—psychosis
perphenazine—psychosis
Persantin—thromboembolic disease
Persantine—thromboembolic disease
phenindione—thromboembolic disease
phenobarbitol—anxiety
phensuximide—seizures
phenylalanine mustard—cancer, lymphoma, leukemia
phenytoin—seizures
pindolol—hypertension, ischemic heart disease

pipotiazine—psychosis
pirbuterol—asthma
Plendil—hypertension, ischemic heart disease
polythiazide—edema
prazepam—anxiety
prazosin—hypertension
prednisone—autoimmune/collagen disease, organ transplantation
Premarin—endocrinopathy, contraception
Primatene—asthma
Prinivil—hypertension
procainamide—cardiac arrhythmia
Procan SR—cardiac arrhythmia
Procardia—hypertension, ischemic heart disease
procaterol—asthma
prochlorperazine—psychosis
Prolixin—psychosis
promazine—psychosis
Promine—cardiac arrhythmia
Pronestyl—cardiac arrhythmia
propafenone—cardiac arrhythmia
propranolol—hypertension, ischemic heart disease
ProSom—anxiety
protamine zinc iletin—endocrinopathy, contraception
protriptyline—depression
Proventil—asthma
Prozac—depression
Prozine-50—psychosis
Purinethol—cancer, lymphoma, leukemia
Pyridamole—thromboembolic disease

Quibron—asthma
Quinaglute—cardiac arrhythmia
Quinalan—cardiac arrhythmia
quinapril—hypertension, ischemic heart disease
Quinate—cardiac arrhythmia
quinestrol—endocrinopathy, contraception
Quinethazone—edema
Quinidex—cardiac arrhythmia
quinidine—cardiac arrhythmia
Quinora—cardiac arrhythmia

ramipril—hypertension
Rauval—psychosis
rauwolfia serpentina—psychosis
Rauzide—psychosis
Regroton—psychosis

Relaxadon—anxiety
Renese—edema
reserpine—psychosis
Rheumatrex—cancer, lymphoma, leukemia
Rythmol—cardiac arrhythmia

salicylic acid—thromboembolic disease
Sandimmune—autoimmune/collagen disease, organ transplantation
secobarbital—anxiety
Seconal—anxiety
Semilente—endocrinopathy, contraception
Ser-Ap-Es—hypertension
Serax—anxiety
Serentil—psychosis
Serpasil—psychosis
Sinequan—depression
Sofarin—thromboembolic disease
Solfoton—anxiety
Solu-Medrol—autoimmune/collagen disease, organ transplantation
Somophyllin—asthma
Sorbitrate—hypertension, ischemic heart disease
Spasmolin—anxiety
Spasmophen—anxiety
spironolactone—edema
Stelazine—psychosis
Stilphostrol—endocrinopathy, contraception
Suprazine—psychosis
Synthroid—endocrinopathy, contraception

talbutal—anxiety
Tambocor—cardiac arrhythmia
Tegretol—seizures
temazepam—anxiety
Tenormin—hypertension, ischemic heart disease
terazosin—hypertension
terbutaline—asthma
Thalitone—edema
Theobid—asthma
Theo-Dur—asthma
Theolair—asthma
theophylline—asthma
Theostat—asthma
thiopropazate—psychosis
thioproperazine—psychosis
thioridazine—psychosis

Thorazine—psychosis
Thylline—asthma
thyroxine—endocrinopathy, contraception
Ticlid—thromboembolic disease
ticlopidine—thromboembolic disease
timolol—hypertension, ischemic heart disease
Tindal—psychosis
tocainide—cardiac arrhythmia
tofranil—depression
Tolamide—endocrinopathy, contraception
tolazamide—endocrinopathy, contraception
tolbutamide—endocrinopathy, contraception
Tolinase—endocrinopathy, contraception
Tonocard—cardiac arrhythmia
Transderm-Nitro—hypertension, ischemic heart disease
Tranxene—anxiety
trazodone—depression
Trialodine—depression
triamcinolone—autoimmune/collagen disease, organ transplantation
triamterene—edema
triazolam—anxiety
trichlormethiazide—edema
Tridil—hypertension, ischemic heart disease
Tridione—seizures
trifluoperazine—psychosis
triflupromazine—psychosis
Trilafon—psychosis
trimethadione—seizures
trimipramine—depression
Tri-Norinyl—endocrinopathy, contraception
Tuinal—anxiety

Ultralente—endocrinopathy, contraception

Valergen—endocrinopathy, contraception
Valium—anxiety
Vapo-Iso—asthma
Vascor—hypertension, ischemic heart disease
Vasotec—hypertension
Velosulin—endocrinopathy, contraception
Ventolin—asthma
verapamil—hypertension, ischemic heart disease
Vesprin—psychosis

warfarin—thromboembolic disease

Xanax—anxiety

Zarontin—seizures
Zaroxolyn—edema
Zestril—hypertension
Zetran—anxiety

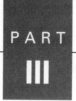

PART

III

Soft Tissue Diseases

SINGLE INTRAORAL SWELLINGS

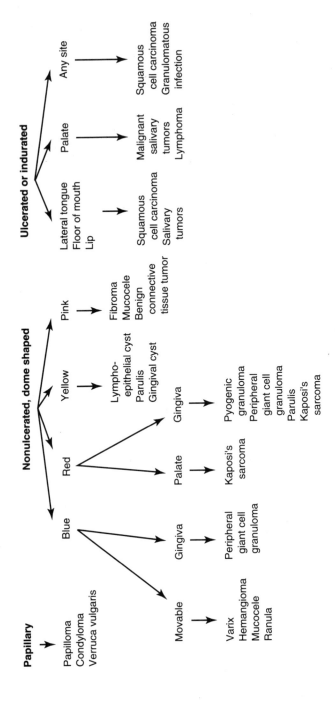

MULTIPLE AND MULTIFOCAL MUCOSAL SWELLINGS

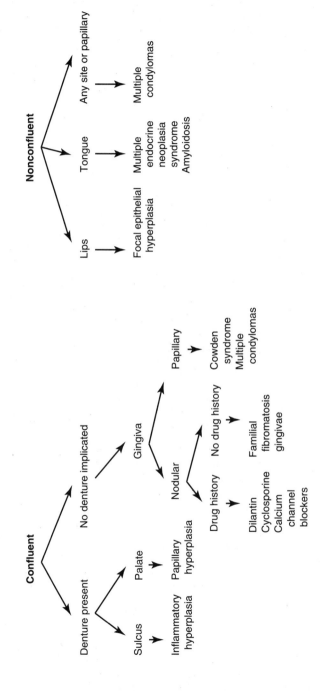

SWELLINGS OF THE FACE AND NECK

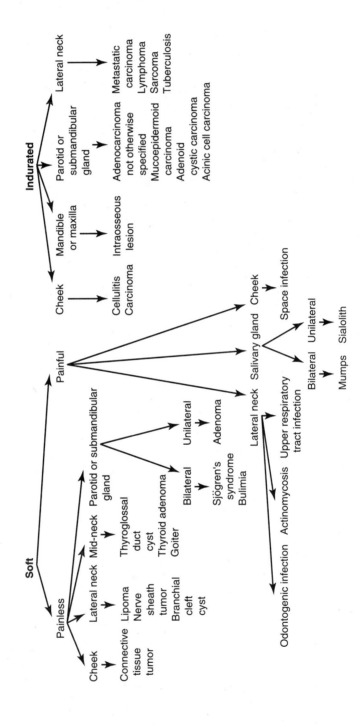

SOFT SWELLINGS OF THE FACE AND NECK

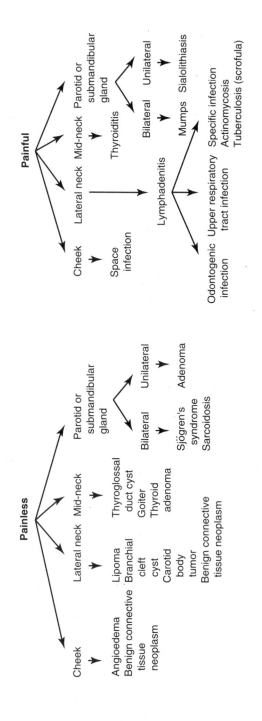

Painless

Cheek → Angioedema, Benign connective tissue neoplasm

Lateral neck → Lipoma, Branchial cleft cyst, Carotid body tumor, Benign connective tissue neoplasm

Mid-neck → Thyroglossal duct cyst, Goiter, Thyroid adenoma

Parotid or submandibular gland
- Bilateral → Sjögren's syndrome, Sarcoidosis
- Unilateral → Adenoma

Painful

Cheek → Space infection

Lateral neck → Lymphadenitis → Odontogenic infection, Upper respiratory tract infection → Specific infection, Actinomycosis, Tuberculosis (scrofula)

Mid-neck → Thyroiditis

Parotid or submandibular gland
- Bilateral → Mumps
- Unilateral → Sialolithiasis

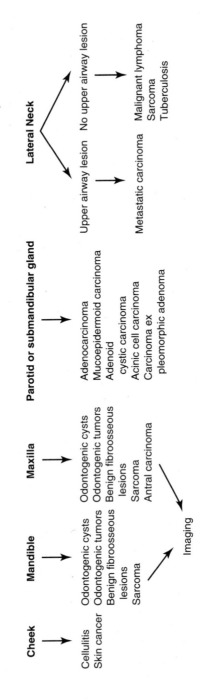

INDURATED SWELLINGS OF THE FACE AND NECK

Cheek

Cellulitis
Skin cancer

Mandible

Odontogenic cysts
Odontogenic tumors
Benign fibroosseous
lesions
Sarcoma

Maxilla

Odontogenic cysts
Odontogenic tumors
Benign fibroosseous
lesions
Sarcoma
Antral carcinoma

Imaging

Parotid or submandibular gland

Adenocarcinoma
Mucoepidermoid carcinoma
Adenoid
cystic carcinoma
Acinic cell carcinoma
Carcinoma ex
pleomorphic adenoma

Lateral Neck

Upper airway lesion

Metastatic carcinoma

No upper airway lesion

Malignant lymphoma
Sarcoma
Tuberculosis

Oral Soft Tissue Swellings by Site

PALATE

Apical abscess
Torus palatinus
Fibrous hyperplasia
Pleomorphic adenoma
Adenoid cystic carcinoma
Mucoepidermoid carcinoma
Polymorphous low-grade adenocarcinoma
Kaposi's sarcoma
Lymphoma

Significant Findings

1. Midline location, indurated, lobulated—torus
2. Associated pain, odontogenic infection—abscess
3. Nonulcerated, off midline—adenoma, hyperplasia
4. Indurated, ulcerated, off midline—adenocarcinoma, lymphoma
5. HIV-positive—lymphoma, Kaposi's sarcoma (particularly if purple)

Diagnostic Procedures

1. Radiographs and endodontic testing are necessary for suspected abscess.
2. Computed tomography can be used to determine bone involvement.
3. Incisional biopsy is appropriate for suspected neoplasms.
4. HIV serotesting should be undertaken for high-risk patients.

Management

1. Odontogenic infection is managed with endodontic therapy or extraction, incision and drainage of abscess, and analgesics and antibiotics if needed
2. Torus requires no treatment but can be surgically excised if it interferes with seating of a dental prosthesis.
3. Conservative surgical excision is appropriate for pleomorphic adenoma and fibrous hyperplasia.
4. Adenocarcinoma should undergo wide excision or radical resection, depending on type and grade of malignancy.
5. Lymphoma requires radiation therapy and chemotherapy.
6. Kaposi's sarcoma requires radiation therapy or sclerotherapy.

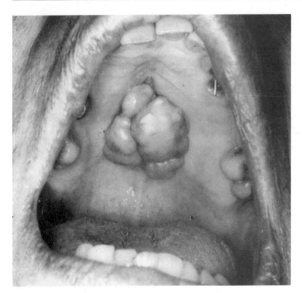

Palatal torus

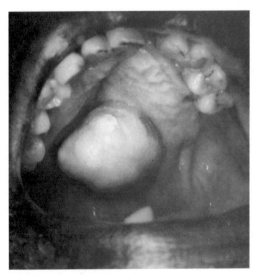

Pleomorphic adenoma

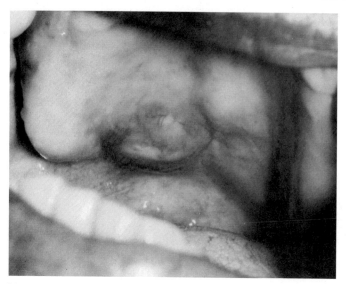

Mucoepidermoid carcinoma

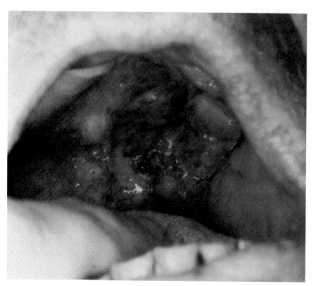

Lymphoma

LOCALIZED GINGIVAL MASSES

Pyogenic granuloma
Peripheral fibroma
Peripheral ossifying fibroma
Peripheral giant cell granuloma
Parulis
Gingival cyst
Neoplasm

Significant Findings

1. Soft and fluctuant with or without drainage—possible infection of pulpal or periodontal origin, resulting in a fistula with parulis
2. Coloration:
   a. Bright red—pyogenic granuloma
   b. Bluish purple—giant cell granuloma
   c. Normal coral pink—peripheral fibroma or ossifying fibroma
   d. Whitish yellow—gingival cyst
3. Pregnancy—pyogenic granuloma, giant cell granuloma, and peripheral ossifying fibroma
4. Location:
   a. Interdental papilla area—usually reactive proliferation
   b. Attached gingiva, below free margin—gingival cyst
   c. Solid focal mass—possibly peripheral odontogenic tumor
   d. Gingival epithelium—predilection for squamous cell carcinoma, lymphoma
   e. Ulcerated, and indurated—squamous cell carcinoma, lymphoma

Diagnostic Procedures

1. Aspiration yields viscous white fluid in gingival cyst; parulis contains a less viscous whitish yellow exudate.
2. Periapical films, pulp testing, and periodontal probing can determine the presence of pulpal or periodontal source of infection.
3. Gingival probing can uncover foreign material entrapped within the sulcus, which may have induced a reactive proliferation.
4. When the aforementioned diagnostic procedures are not productive, a biopsy should be performed. This biopsy should be taken down to the periosteum.

Management

1. Reactive proliferations should be completely excised, with thorough root planing and curettage. Giant cell lesions and peripheral ossifying fibroma arise from periosteal and periodontal ligament (PDL) cells and therefore require deep surgical excision into the PDL or subperiosteal dissection.
2. Odontogenic cyst and tumors require surgical excision.

3. For odontogenic and periodontal infections, the infectious source must be treated (e.g., root canal therapy, apicoectomy, periodontal surgery).

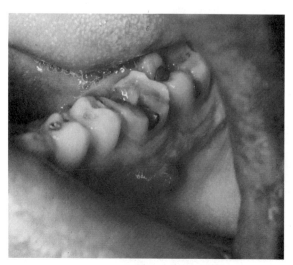

Parulis

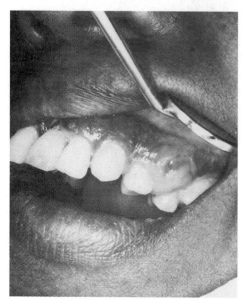

Peripheral ossifying fibroma

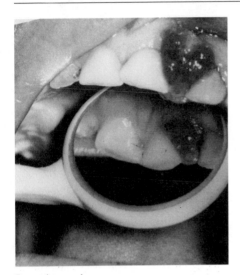

Pyogenic granuloma

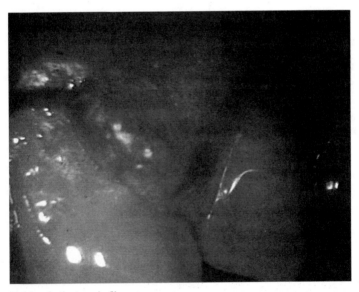

Peripheral odontogenic fibroma

GENERALIZED OR DIFFUSE GINGIVAL SWELLINGS

Drug-induced
Hyperplastic gingivitis, nonspecific
Leukemia
Fibromatosis gingivae

Significant Findings

1. History of use of a drug that causes gingival enlargement—phenytoin, calcium channel blockers, or cyclosporine.
2. Family history of gingival enlargement is significant for familial fibromatosis gingivae, an extremely rare disease.
3. Hormonal changes occurring during pregnancy and puberty in females are thought to influence an exaggerated hyperplastic gingival response to plaque.
4. By history and physical examination, weakness, malaise, tiredness, pallor, and purpura suggest leukemia. Gingival enlargement occurs in fewer than 10% of patients with leukemia.

Diagnostic Procedures

1. A complete blood count should be ordered to detect leukemia in patients with no other known predisposing factors for gingival enlargement and in patients with physical signs suggestive of leukemia.
2. Incisional biopsy discloses a leukemic infiltrate.

Management

1. Withdrawal of medications responsible for the enlargement results in diminution but not total resolution of swelling. More often, the medications are essential to the management of the medical condition and cannot be decreased. Gingivectomy with scaling, curettage, and intensive home care maintenance usually minimizes the drug effects on the gingiva.
2. Leukemia requires referral to a medical oncologist or hematologist. With appropriate treatment, the gingival swelling decreases.
3. The fibrotic swellings of genetic disease are difficult to manage. Periodic gingivectomies are usually requested by the patient for cosmetic reasons. The enlargement does not necessarily predispose to apical migration of the gingival attachment.
4. Hyperplastic gingivitis associated with hormonal changes in women dramatically diminishes once the imbalance has self-corrected, as in termination of pregnancy or passage through puberty. In both instances, gingival enlargements may require surgical recontouring.

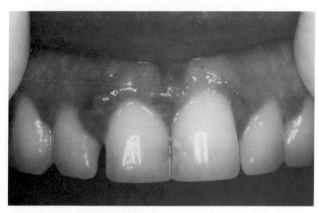

Hyperplastic gingivitis

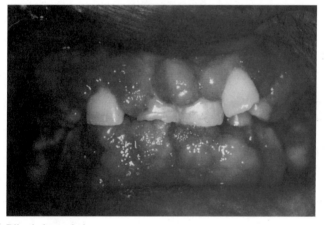

Dilantin hyperplasia

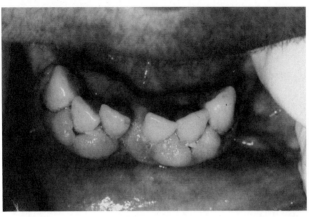

Nifedipine hyperplasia

BUCCAL AND LIP MUCOSA

Fibrous hyperplasia (fibroma)
Mesenchymal neoplasm
Mucocele
Squamous cell carcinoma
Verrucous carcinoma
Salivary neoplasm

Significant Findings

1. Smooth surface, dome-shaped along occlusal plane—fibroma
2. Soft and fluctuant on lip—mucocele
3. Movable and firm submucosal mass—mesenchymal neoplasm (e.g., lipoma, nerve sheath tumor) or benign salivary tumor (e.g., pleomorphic adenoma, monomorphic adenoma, including basal cell and canalicular variants)
4. Indurated or ulcerated—carcinoma, adenocarcinoma
5. White, verrucous or papillary—verrucous carcinoma

Diagnostic Procedures

1. Aspiration of suspected mucoceles obtains white mucoid contents.
2. Excisional biopsy is recommended for all nodular smooth masses.
3. Incisional biopsy is advisable for suspected carcinomas and large nonencapsulated submucosal masses.

Management

1. Local excision or enucleation is appropriate for fibroma, benign mesenchymal neoplasms, and salivary adenomas.
2. Mucoceles should be excised and the underlying feeder minor salivary glands removed.
3. Verrucous carcinoma requires wide local excision with tumor-free margins. Squamous cell carcinoma and salivary adenocarcinoma can be treated with wide surgical excision, radiotherapy, or combined therapy. A clinical and imaging workup for possible metastatic disease is required for malignancies.

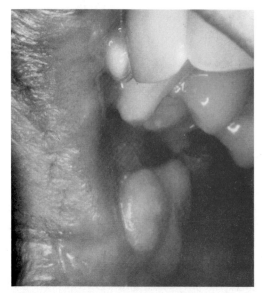

Fibrous hyperplasia

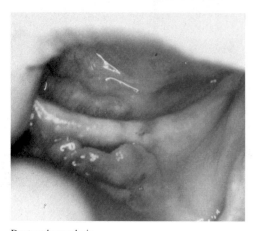

Denture hyperplasia

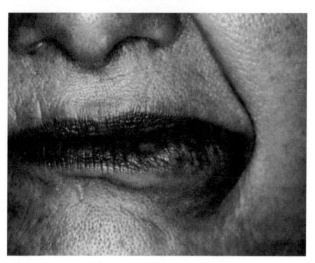

Hemangioma of lower lip

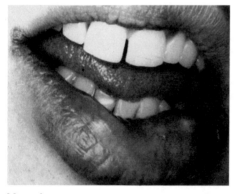

Mucocele

DORSAL AND LATERAL TONGUE

Fibrous hyperplasia (fibroma)
Hyperplastic lingual tonsil
Granular cell tumor
Mesenchymal neoplasm
Squamous cell carcinoma

Significant Findings

1. Nonulcerated submucosal nodules usually represent benign reactive lesions and connective tissue tumors (e.g., fibromas, neural sheath neoplasms, granular cell tumors).
2. Depapillation with yellow discoloration is suggestive of granular cell tumor.
3. Multinodular, nonulcerated soft swellings at the lateral border of the tongue base junction are consistent with hyperplastic tonsillar tissue (foliate papillitis).
4. Induration and ulceration with surrounding leukoplakia or erythroplakia should arouse suspicion of malignancy, particularly in tobacco users.
5. Dorsal tongue racemose multinodular masses suggest vascular tumors. If the lesions are blue or red, hemangioma is likely; if they are yellowish, lymphangioma is suggested.

Diagnostic Procedures

1. When hyperplastic lingual tonsil is suspected, periodic follow-up is recommended. Any increase in size, induration, or ulceration warrants biopsy.
2. Excisional biopsy is recommended for small lesions, incisional biopsy for larger masses.

Management

1. Benign connective tissue neoplasms, including granular cell tumors, and reactive fibrous hyperplasias, vascular tumors excepted, rarely recur after complete surgical excision.
2. Hemangiomas and lymphangiomas can be treated by excision or sclerotherapy in adults. Many such tumors extend deeply into the intrinsic muscles of the tongue, and only debulking is required for functional and cosmetic purposes. Nearly 90% of childhood vascular hamartomas resolve or involute spontaneously during or after puberty. Therefore, after diagnostic biopsy, periodic follow-up without treatment is recommended until the patient reaches adulthood.

3. Squamous cell carcinoma is treated by surgery, radiotherapy, or combined therapy. A clinical and imaging workup for possible metastatic disease is required for malignancies.

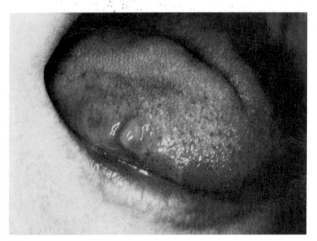

Fibroma

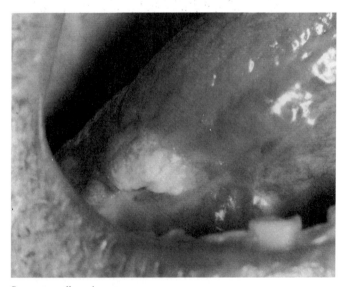

Squamous cell carcinoma

FLOOR OF MOUTH AND VENTRAL TONGUE

Ranula (mucocele)
Dermoid cyst
Lymphoepithelial cyst and ectopic tonsil
Salivary neoplasm
Squamous cell carcinoma

Significant Findings

1. A soft fluctuant lesion in the oral floor, off the midline, suggests a ranula, whereas a soft fluctuant or doughy submucosal mass in the midline oral floor suggests a dermoid cyst.
2. Small single or racemose clustered submucosal masses with yellow coloration are consistent with lymphoid aggregates, some of which may be cystic.
3. Salivary tumors can be benign or malignant, arising from the minor salivary glands of the oral floor and ventral tongue or from the sublingual gland. Movability suggests benignity; induration and fixation are more consistent with adenocarcinoma. Malignant salivary tumors are more common than benign ones in the sublingual gland.
4. Induration, ulceration, and surrounding erythema or leukoplakia suggest squamous cancer.

Diagnostic Procedures

1. Aspiration yields milky or clear fluid from a ranula. Because dermoid cysts contain keratin, either nothing can be aspirated or thick white caseous material is evident.
2. Incisional biopsy is recommended for large lesions, excisional biopsy for small masses.

Management

1. Ranulas should be treated by enucleation of the cystic mass and its surrounding capsule. Since these are large mucoceles and rarely have an epithelial lining, marsupialization is not usually indicated.
2. Simple excision or enucleation is sufficient for benign submucosal lesions, including hyperplastic and cystic lymphoid aggregates.
3. Dermoid cysts may lie above or below the mylohyoid muscle. If they lie above, an intraoral approach with enucleation is recommended. If they lie below, either an intraoral or extraoral approach can be taken.
4. Benign salivary tumors arising deep in the sublingual gland require excision with sialectomy.
5. Squamous cell carcinoma and salivary adenocarcinomas are treated by wide surgical excision, with or without combined radiotherapy. Imaging studies should be performed to rule out local

invasion of the mandible, as well as to determine the presence of pulmonary or regional nodal metastases.

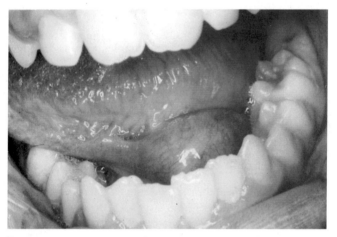

Ranula

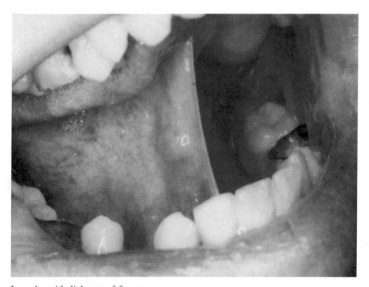

Lymphoepithelial cyst of frenum

Extraoral Soft Tissue Swellings by Site

PAROTID REGION

Endemic parotitis
Sjögren's syndrome
Sialolithiasis or sialadenitis
Adenoma
    Pleomorphic adenoma
    Monomorphic adenoma
    Papillary cystadenoma lymphomatosum (Warthin's tumor)
Adenocarcinoma
    Adenoid cystic carcinoma
    Mucoepidermoid carcinoma
    Acinic cell carcinoma
Mesenchymal neoplasm

Significant Findings

1. Diffuse bilateral swelling is encountered in mumps and Sjögren's syndrome, whereas focal bilateral nodules are occasionally seen in Warthin's tumors. Endemic parotitis is usually a childhood infection, and there is accompanying fever and malaise. In Sjögren's syndrome, xerostomia, xerophthalmia, and rheumatoid arthritis can occur simultaneously. Bilateral Warthin's tumors occur in the elderly.
2. Unilateral parotid masses in a child are probably benign mesenchymal tumors (e.g., cellular hemangioma, fibrous histiocytoma, or xanthogranuloma).
3. Soft and movable masses most likely represent benign adenomas, pleomorphic adenoma being most common. Elderly men are more prone to have papillary cystadenoma lymphomatosum; elderly women develop oncocytoma.
4. Fixed and indurated swellings are likely to represent adenocarcinoma, and facial nerve palsy is invariably a sign of malignancy when a parotid mass is detected.

Diagnostic Procedures

1. Elevated temperature and parotid pain suggest mumps. Elevated levels of serum amylase support the diagnosis.
2. Fine-needle aspiration cytology often yields a definitive diagnosis of neoplastic processes. Open biopsy is not recommended because of its propensity to cause extracapsular seeding and spread.
3. In suspected Sjögren's syndrome, a lower lip biopsy for lymphoid infiltrate focal scores is recommended (1+ being suggestive, 2+ to 4+ being highly supportive) along with autoantibody assessments for rheumatoid factor, SS-Rho, and SS-La. A parotid tail biopsy

for detection of benign lymphoepithelial lesion can also be undertaken.

4. Magnetic resonance imaging and computed tomography are often diagnostic and can disclose the extent of disease. A panoramic film can reveal the presence of a parotid duct sialolith.

Management

1. Mumps is treated by bed rest, nutritional support, and analgesics. Care should be taken to prevent gonadal extension.

2. Sjögren's syndrome is a management dilemma because the dryness is irreversible. Pilocarpine therapy may be of benefit early on, and transglossal electrical stimulation devices may stimulate salivation. Artificial saliva preparations and meticulous dental hygiene procedures with daily topical fluoride treatments must be instituted to prevent root caries.

3. Stones should be removed manually or surgically. If salivary function fails to return, parotidectomy should be considered in an effort to prevent retrograde bacterial acute sialadenitis.

4. Most benign adenomas are treated by lobectomy in continuity with tumor.

5. Malignant tumors are treated in accordance with grade of malignancy. Most require parotidectomy. Facial nerve isolation is usually required, and partial or complete temporal bone resection may be necessary. A metastatic workup is required and neck dissection must be performed when clinical or imaging evidence of node metastasis is uncovered.

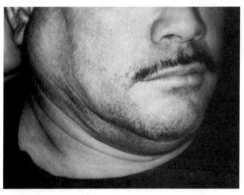

Parotid sialadenitis

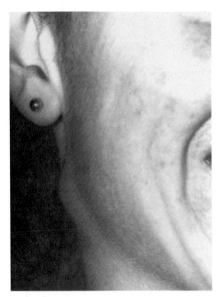

Pleomorphic adenoma

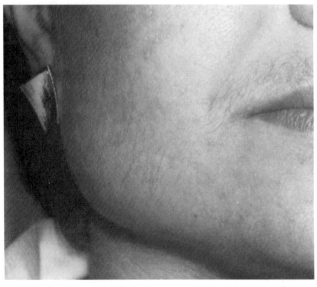

Adenocarcinoma

LATERAL NECK

Branchial cleft cyst
Lymphadenitis
Specific granulomatous inflammation
Carotid body tumor (chemodectoma)
Mesenchymal neoplasm
Metastatic carcinoma
Lymphoma

Significant Findings

1. Soft, movable masses are benign neoplasms or inflammatory lymph nodes: If the mass is fluctuant, branchial cleft cyst is most probable. If it is tender or painful, an inflammatory lesion of the lymph nodes is most likely. If the mass is movable laterally but not vertically, chemodectoma should be considered.
2. Indurated and fixed nodes should arouse suspicion of metastatic carcinoma or lymphoma. A search of the upper airway for a possible primary squamous cell carcinoma should be undertaken. A lateral neck mass in a teenager with ipsilateral hearing loss is suspicious for nasopharyngeal carcinoma.
3. Persistent or progressive swelling, particularly in an adult, that is associated with periodic fever and night sweats without any source of lymphadenopathy should arouse suspicion of lymphoma.
4. Soft tender masses usually indicate lymphadenitis. An infectious source of dental, periodontal, or upper respiratory infection should be investigated.

Diagnostic Procedures

1. A complete head and neck physical examination should be performed to explore for infectious and neoplastic sources of cervical lymphadenopathy.
2. Fine-needle aspiration cytologic examination is appropriate. Open biopsy is recommended only for lesions with a benign appearance clinically (i.e., soft and movable).
3. Magnetic resonance imaging and dental radiography should be performed.

Management

1. For lymphadenopathy, the infectious source must be eliminated.
2. Mesenchymal neoplasms such as lipoma and nerve sheath tumors, as well as chemodectomas, are treated by complete local excision, the latter with presurgical embolization.
3. Lymphomas are managed by combination radiation and chemotherapy, the regimen depending on the histologic diagnosis and stage of disease.

4. Metastatic carcinoma is treated by surgery, radiation therapy, or combined therapy to include the primary lesion.

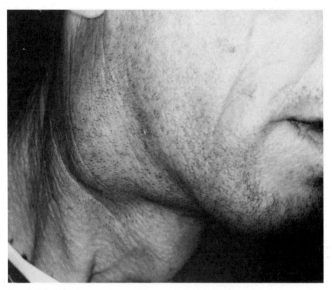

Branchial cleft cyst

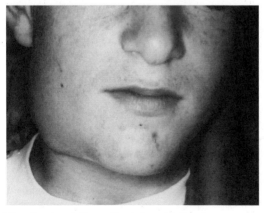

Granulomatous inflammation (cat scratch fever)

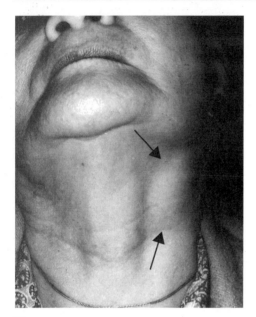

Lipoma

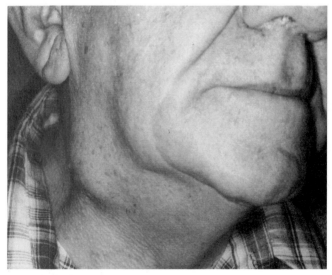

Metastatic carcinoma

MIDLINE NECK

Goiter
Thyroiditis
Thyroglossal cyst
Thyroid adenoma
Thyroid carcinoma

Significant Findings

1. Multinodular enlargements are usually forms of goiter.
2. Focal thyroid nodules can be benign or malignant.
3. Diffuse thyroid enlargements represent forms of goiter or thyroiditis. If painful, subacute viral thyroiditis is probable.
4. If a mass is located above the thyroid, in the flexure of the anterior neck over the hyoid, thyroglossal duct cyst is most likely.

Diagnostic Procedures

1. Thyroid function tests should be ordered for thyroid enlargements to include T_3, T_4, and thyroid-stimulating hormone.
2. Magnetic resonance imaging can be diagnostic, especially for nodular goiter. Radio-iodine uptake is also useful: hot nodules are benign, whereas cold nodules are suggestive of malignancy.
3. Fine-needle aspiration cytology is indicated over biopsy as an initial diagnostic screening analysis.

Management

1. Euthyroid goiter can be left untreated, or a partial thyroidectomy can be performed.
2. Hyperthyroidism with goiter (Graves' disease) is managed surgically or by radioisotope therapy. Hypothyroidism should be treated medically.
3. Benign adenomas are treated by subtotal thyroidectomy.
4. Thyroglossal duct cyst is treated by surgical excision, and removal of the hyoid bone may be required.
5. Thyroid carcinomas are generally treated by total thyroidectomy.

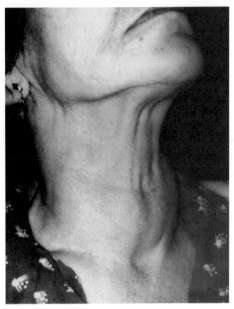

Goiter

FOCAL FACIAL SKIN NODULES

Sebaceous cyst
Intradermal nevus
Seborrheic keratosis
Keratoacanthoma
Basal cell carcinoma
Squamous cell carcinoma
Adnexal skin tumors

Significant Findings

1. Location:
   a. Upper lip and face—basal cell carcinoma
   b. Lower lip—squamous cell carcinoma
   c. Malar eminence region—nodular melanoma
2. Appearance:
   a. Brown, crusted, ulcerated—carcinoma with blood pigment
   b. Smooth and nonulcerated—nevus
   c. Waxy yellowish brown—seborrheic keratosis
   d. Pearly white with telangiectasia—nevus or basal cell carcinoma
   e. Black—nevus, melanoma
3. Configuration:
   a. Crateriform with central plug—keratoacanthoma, basal cell carcinoma, or squamous cell carcinoma
   b. Pasted-on appearance—seborrheic keratosis
   c. Movable subdermal nodule—sebaceous cyst
4. Duration:
   a. Present for many years without any change in size—nevus
   b. History of progressive increase in size—malignancy
   c. History of relatively rapid growth followed by cessation of growth—seborrheic keratosis and keratoacanthoma

Diagnostic Procedure

Incisional biopsy for large lesions, excisional biopsy for smaller masses.

Management

1. Benign lesions—including seborrheic keratoses, sebaceous cysts, nevi, benign adnexal skin tumors, and keratoacanthomas—are treated by simple excision.
2. Basal and squamous cell carcinomas are treated by wide local excision, Mohs chemosurgery, and by radiation therapy. In squamous cell carcinoma, a workup for local and distant metastases is required. If neck nodes are palpated or found on imaging, neck dissection, radiation, or both may be required. Rare malignant adnexal skin tumors are treated by wide local excision.

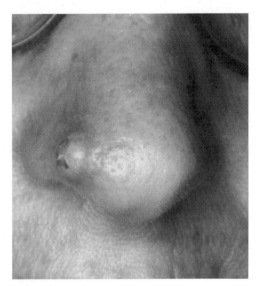

Basal cell carcinoma

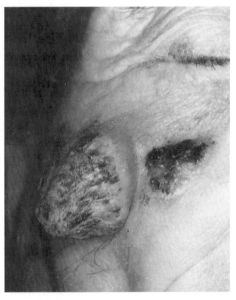

Keratoacanthoma

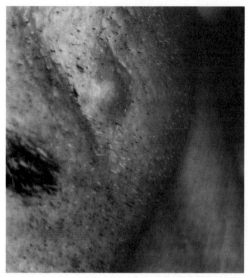

Sebaceous cyst

DIFFUSE FACIAL SWELLINGS

Angioneurotic edema
Cellulitis
Space infection
Soft tissue emphysema
Cheilitis granulomatosa

Significant Findings

1. Associated pain symptoms and fever indicate spread of infection, usually odontogenic in origin. Induration is consistent with cellulitis, fluctuation with space infection.
2. Soft, painless swellings are noninfectious, such as angioedema (particularly if pruritic) or air emphysema (particularly if crepitant).
3. Swelling that is localized to the lips and multinodular is cheilitis granulomatosa; if it is homogeneous and soft, it is angioedema.
4. History of air introduction into soft tissues, particularly from air or water syringe, indicates soft tissue emphysema.
5. Allergy history, familial involvement, or recurrent swellings tend to indicate angioedema.

Diagnostic Procedures

1. Radiographs and endodontic testing are required for suspected odontogenic infections.
2. Inflammatory swellings can be incised and drained to explore for purulent exudate. Culture and sensitivity testing is also in order.
3. Lip enlargements should undergo biopsy for suspected granulomatous inflammation.
4. C1–esterase inhibitor can be assayed for suspected familial angioedema.

Management

1. For angioneurotic edema, any persistent allergens should be withdrawn and antihistamines and systemic steroids prescribed.
2. Incision and drainage are necessary for space infections, as are use of topical hot packs, antibiotic therapy, and endodontic treatment or extraction if nonrestorable.
3. Incision and drainage and antibiotic prophylaxis are appropriate for air emphysema.
4. Intralesional steroid injections and cosmetic surgery in conjunction with steroids may be necessary for cheilitis granulomatosa.

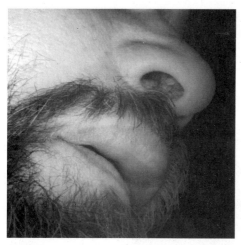

Angioedema

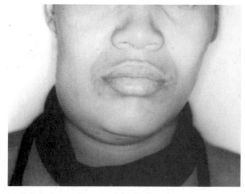

Cellulitis from odontogenic infection

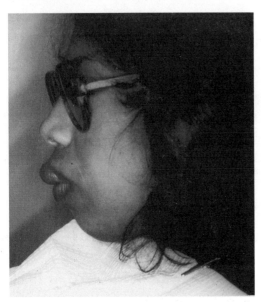

Cheilitis granulomatosa

Oral Soft Tissue Swellings by Clinical Features

SMOOTH, DOME-SHAPED

Traumatic and peripheral fibroma
Peripheral ossifying fibroma
Herniated buccal fat pad
Mucocele
Mesenchymal neoplasms

Significant Findings

1. A history of trauma or irritation is often obtained for traumatic fibroma, herniated fat pad, and mucoceles.
2. Mucoceles are soft and fluctuant; herniated fat pads are also soft and flabby but not fluctuant. The others in this group vary from soft to firm.
3. Peripheral fibroma and ossifying fibroma arise from the attached gingiva, usually at the level of the interdental papilla. Herniated fat pad is found in the buccal mucosa. Fibromas and mucoceles are most often encountered on the lower lip, mandibular vestibule, and buccal mucosa. Nerve sheath tumors and granular cell tumors are usually noted on the tongue and in the buccal mucosa as firm swellings.

Diagnostic Procedure

For all of these entities, the diagnosis is based on histopathologic features. Biopsy is therefore recommended for all smooth, dome-shaped lesions.

Management

1. Local excision is the treatment of choice for all lesions in this group. Gingival proliferations require adjunctive root planing in order to eliminate irritants. Mucoceles should be excised in conjunction with the feeder glands located at the base.
2. Herniated buccal fat pad can usually be diagnosed at the time of surgery since the tissue is lobulated and yellow. In these instances, excision should be accompanied by closure of any split or severance of the buccinator muscle through which the fat pad has extruded.

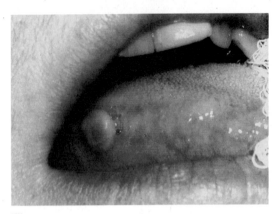

Fibroma

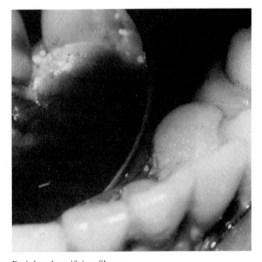

Peripheral ossifying fibroma

SINGLE PAPILLARY

Squamous papilloma
Condyloma
Verruca vulgaris
Sialadenoma papilliferum
Verruciform xanthoma

Significant Findings

1. Papillary swellings that are focal and localized to mucosa are most likely benign papillomas.
2. Multiple and clustered papillary swellings are suggestive of condyloma and may have been transmitted by orogenital contact. A condyloma can also be a single, large, sessile lesion. A history of orogenital contact may be relevant.
3. Papillary and verrucous masses of the lip vermilion are most likely common warts (verruca vulgaris).
4. Papillary masses in the palate may involve salivary ducts, being sialadenomas.
5. White verrucous lesions of the gingiva or palate may be verruciform xanthomas, particularly if they have a yellowish cast.

Diagnostic Procedures

1. Biopsy should be undertaken—excisional for small defined lesions, incisional for diffuse or multifocal papillary masses.
2. DNA in situ hybridization can be useful in identification of human papillomavirus. Human papillomaviruses 6 and 11 are seen in papillomas and condylomas; human papillomaviruses 2 and 4 are present in verruca vulgaris.

Management

1. Focal lesions can be treated by excisional biopsy or laser surgery.
2. Multiple papillomas, as encountered in condylomas, are difficult to eradicate since they tend to recur. Laser surgery is the treatment of choice.

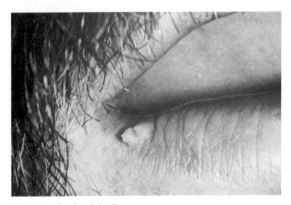

Verruca vulgaris of the lip

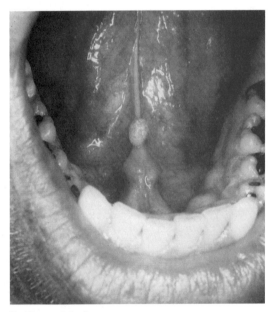

Papilloma of the frenum

MULTIPLE PAPILLARY OR MULTINODULAR

Condyloma acuminatum
Papillary hyperplasia
Proliferative verrucous leukoplakia
Papillary and verrucous forms of carcinoma
Syndrome-associated papillomatosis

Significant Findings

1. Multiple confluent papillary lesions of the gingiva, lips, and tongue, appearing as isolated papillomas with intervening normal mucosa suggest venereal warts (condyloma). A history of orogenital contact is significant.
2. Confinement to the palatal vault under a full denture is consistent with papillomatosis or papillary hyperplasia.
3. Diffuse papillary lesions with a white verrucous surface in older patients, involving the gingiva, alveolus, and buccal mucosa or vestibule suggest proliferative verrucous leukoplakia, a precancerous lesion. Only half of these people smoke or use smokeless tobacco.
4. Extensive diffuse white and red papillary lesions, particularly those more than 2 cm in diameter, suggest verrucous carcinoma or papillary forms of squamous cell carcinoma.
5. Diffuse and multifocal oral papillary lesions occur as components of two syndromes:
   a. Cowden syndrome —oral papillary lesions, cutaneous nodules and cysts, thyroid enlargement, breast tumors
   b. Focal dermal hypoplasia—oral and labial papillomas, doughy cutaneous nodular masses of herniated subcutaneous connective tissues.
6. In multiple endocrine neoplasia syndrome, the oral lesions are multiple papules or nodules rather than papillomas. This syndrome is characterized by multiple oral, labial, and conjunctival neuromatous papules, thyroid medullary carcinoma, and adrenal pheochromocytoma.

Diagnostic Procedures

1. Biopsy is recommended for all these lesions.
2. DNA in situ hybridization can disclose the papillomavirus genotype.
3. Complete physical examination should be undertaken for suspected syndrome-related papillary lesions.

Management

1. Laser and conventional surgery can be used to excise condylomas and papillary hyperplasia.

2. Wide excision is required for proliferative verrucous leukoplakia and verrucous carcinoma, although recurrence is common. Close periodic follow-up is essential.
3. Papillary squamous carcinoma requires wide excision; lymph node metastasis, although rare, does occur.
4. Suspected Cowden syndrome or focal dermal hypoplasia involves other tissue. A dermatology consultation is recommended.
5. A diagnosis of multiple endocrine neoplasia requires a workup for endocrine tumors that may be potentially fatal, and surgical intervention should be performed as soon as possible.

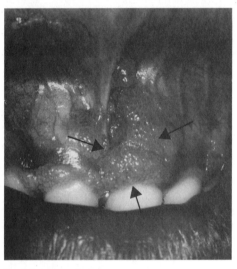

Condyloma acuminatum

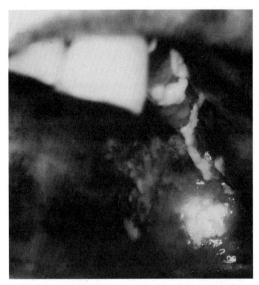

Proliferative verrucous leukoplakia

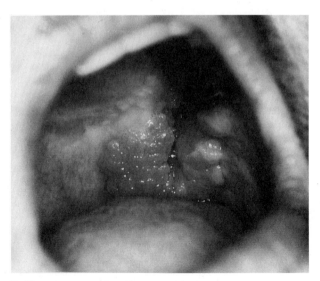

Papillary squamous cell carcinoma

SOFT AND FLUCTUANT SUBMUCOSAL AND SUBDERMAL MASSES

Dermoid cyst
Ranula
Thyroglossal cyst
Lingual thyroid nodule
Gastric cyst
Nasoalveolar cyst
Cyst of the incisive papilla
Branchial cleft cyst
Lipoma
Lymphangioma
Hemangioma

Significant Findings

1. Most of these masses are cysts that arise from embryonic epithelial remnants, and they are therefore localized to a specific site:
   a. Anterior midline floor of mouth—dermoid cyst
   b. Lateral aspect of the floor of mouth—ranula
   c. Midline tongue base or suprathyroid neck—thyroglossal duct cyst
   d. Midline tongue base—lingual thyroid nodule (undescended thyroid)
   e. Tongue—gastric cyst
   f. Maxillary labial fold or ala of nose region—nasoalveolar cyst
   g. Incisive papilla—cyst of the incisive papilla
   h. Lateral neck—branchial cleft cyst
2. A doughy consistency indicates a dermoid cyst.

Diagnostic Procedures

1. Clear yellow fluid can be aspirated from most cysts, ranulas, and lymphangiomas. Blood is seen with hemangiomas; thick white aspirate indicates a dermoid cyst.
2. Magnetic resonance imaging can disclose the extent of a mass, and imaging characteristics may be diagnostic.
3. Biopsy, usually by excision, is recommended.
4. If a cold compress induces firmness, lipoma is suggested.

Management

1. Cysts, ranulas, lipomas, and localized vascular tumors are managed by surgical enucleation and excision.
2. Sclerosing agents are an option for vascular tumors.

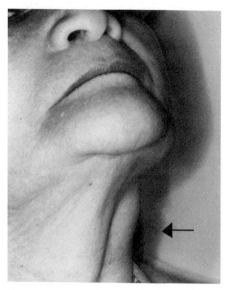

Lipoma

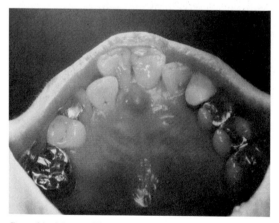

Cyst of incisive papilla

DEEP AND FIRM SUBMUCOSAL AND SUBDERMAL MASSES

Fibromatosis
Mesenchymal tumor
Sarcoma

Significant Findings

1. Deep palpable masses that are diffuse and not well delineated may be sarcomas or fibromatosis.
2. Deep, movable or encapsulated, firm masses are most likely benign mesenchymal tumors, such as nerve sheath tumors, lipomas, or fibrous histiocytomas.

Diagnostic Procedures

1. Only biopsy can yield a definitive diagnosis. Most such lesions are large, so excisional biopsy is untenable. Fine-needle aspiration cytology is recommended for deep-seated firm masses, since open biopsy can disseminate a malignant tumor, particularly if it turns out to be a metastatic node.
2. Deep-seated connective tissue lesions may require immunocytochemcial staining to obtain a definitive diagnosis.

Management

1. Fibromatoses are reactive, yet aggressive, fibroblastic proliferations that require wide, complete local excision.
2. Most benign connective tissue tumors are well localized and can be removed by conservative local excision.
3. Sarcomas have a high propensity for hematogenous metastases and must be treated by radical excision. Some types of sarcomas can be managed by combined surgery and chemotherapy.

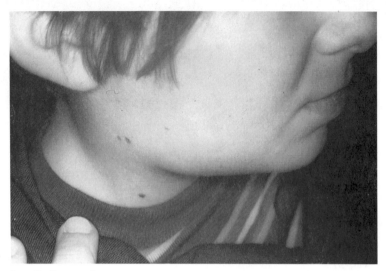

Juvenile fibromatosis

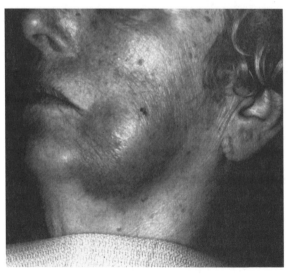

Sarcoma

INDURATED OR ULCERATED MASSES

Benign fibrotic lesion
Squamous cell carcinoma
Adenocarcinoma
Lymphoma
Sarcoma

Significant Findings

1. Some benign processes can show ulceration and be indurated, particularly fibromas and peripheral ossifying fibromas of the gingiva. Most indurated lesions, however, represent a malignant process.
2. Palatal location suggests salivary adenocarcinoma or lymphoma.
3. Lateral tongue, alveolar ridge, and floor of mouth presentation suggests squamous cancer.
4. Sarcomas are extremely rare but can occur anywhere in the oral soft tissues.

Diagnostic Procedures

1. Incisional biopsy is the diagnostic procedure of choice for all indurated or ulcerated masses.
2. For those that occur on or adjacent to bony structures of the palate or alveolar bone, radiographs or other images should be obtained.

Management

1. All malignant neoplasms require aggressive therapy, which is guided by the diagnosis. Squamous cancer is generally treated by combined surgery and radiation, with lymph node dissection or neck irradiation when regional metastases are detected clinically or by magnetic resonance imaging.
2. Most salivary adenocarcinomas are treated by wide surgical excision of tumor and adjacent bone.
3. Sarcomas are treated by surgery; some are managed with combination chemotherapy.
4. Lymphomas are treated by radiation and chemotherapy.
5. In all instances of malignancy, pulmonary films and local imaging studies are required to search for metastases and determine extent of disease.

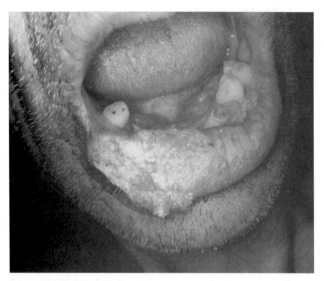

Squamous cell carcinoma

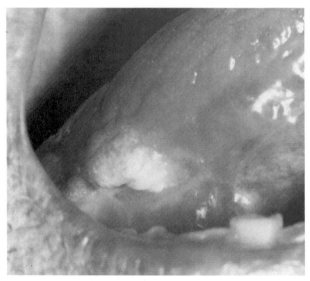

Squamous cell carcinoma

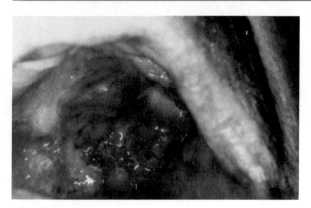

Palatal lymphoma

YELLOW NODULES

Lipoma
Lymphoepithelial cyst
Lymphangioma
Granular cell tumor
Gingival cyst
Fordyce's granules

Significant Findings

1. Location:
   a. Buccal mucosa—lipoma
   b. Tongue—lymphangioma
   c. Floor of the mouth and ventral tongue—lymphoepithelial cyst
   d. Dorsum, lateral tongue and soft palate—granular cell tumor
   e. Buccal mucosa—Fordyce's granules
   f. Attached gingiva, usually the facial aspect in the premolar region—gingival cyst
2. Lymphangiomas are often racemose, and lymphoepithelial cysts may be lobulated.
3. Fordyce's granules are generally multiple but some are large and focal.
4. A radiograph often shows a coin-shaped radiolucency under gingival cysts indicative of the cupping bony erosion common in this lesion.

Diagnostic Procedures

1. Aspiration for suspected gingival cyst yields yellow fluid or white keratinaceous or caseous material.
2. Excisional biopsy is required for the diagnosis of most of these entities.

Management

Surgical exicision is recommended for all yellow nodules except Fordyce's granules, which need no treatment.

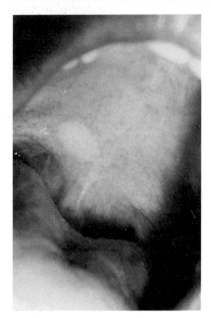

Soft palate granular cell tumor

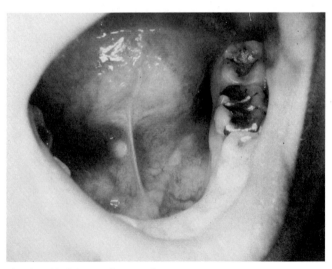

Lymphoepithelial cyst adjacent to frenum

BLACK, BROWN, AND GRAY SWELLINGS

Nevus
Pigmented neuroectodermal tumor of infancy
Melanoma

Significant Findings

1. Focal pigmentations that are raised are usually compound or intramucosal nevi.
2. Diffuse macular pigmentations mixed with nodular swellings, particularly of the anterior maxillary gingiva or anterior palate in adults, are highly suggestive of melanoma.
3. A focal pigmented mass of the anterior maxilla in neonates, along with an associated maxillary radiolucency exhibiting irregular margins, is most often a pigmented neuroectodermal tumor.

Diagnostic Procedures

1. A biopsy is required for all pigmented nodules.
2. Radiographs should be obtained to search for osseous erosion or a central radiolucency when the lesion overlies bone.
3. In an infant with suspected neuroectodermal tumor, urinary catecholamine metabolites should be investigated, since such tumors secrete these metabolites.

Management

1. Nevi are treated by excision.
2. Melanomas require radical surgical excision of mucosa and underlying bone. Neck dissection may also be included. The prognosis is extremely poor for patients with oral melanoma.
3. Neuroectodermal tumor of infancy is usually benign. Total excision with curettage of the underlying resorbed bone is required, and any developing teeth in continuity with the tumor should be removed.

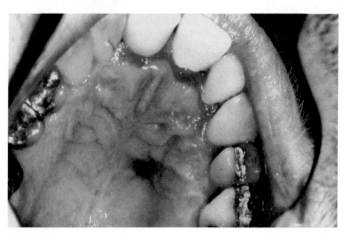

Blue nevus

RED, BLUE, AND PURPLE FOCAL SWELLINGS

Pyogenic granuloma
Peripheral giant cell granuloma
Hemangioma
Varix
Ecchymosis and hematoma
Kaposi's sarcoma
Mucocele or ranula

Significant Findings

1. Blanching:
   a. Lesions that blanch under pressure are usually vascular.
   b. Thrombosed varices, hemorrhage into a mucocele, and extravasated blood in a zone of ecchymosis will not blanch.
2. Location:
   a. Hemangiomas are most common on the tongue as racemose multinodular masses.
   b. Varices, ecchymoses, and mucoceles are most often located on the lip.
   c. Kaposi's sarcomas and the reactive granulomas are seen on the gingiva; the former also tends to arise on the palate.

Diagnostic Procedures

1. If there is a history of bleeding or bruising, a hemorrhagic diathesis must be investigated. Ecchymoses are more often seen with coagulopathies as opposed to platelet disorders, which usually lead to petechiae. Therefore, the first tests to be performed are evaluations of the extrinsic pathway (prothrombin time) and the intrinsic pathway (partial thromboplastin time).
2. These entities (ecchymosis excepted) require biopsy for diagnosis.

Management

1. Pyogenic granuloma and peripheral giant cell granuloma require surgical excision and thorough root planing.
2. Localized varices and hemorrhagic mucoceles are treated by surgical excision.
3. A blood dyscrasia as revealed by prolonged prothrombin or partial thromboplastin time requires a diagnostic workup by a hematologist before treatment can be prescribed.
4. Kaposi's sarcoma lesions respond to low-dose radiation therapy and can be eliminated by injection of sclerosing agents or *Vinca* alkaloids.

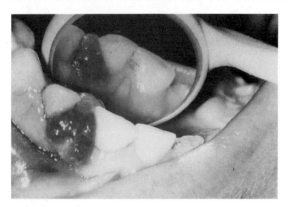

Pyogenic granuloma

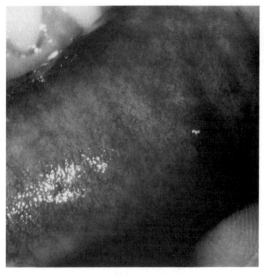

Varix of the lower lip

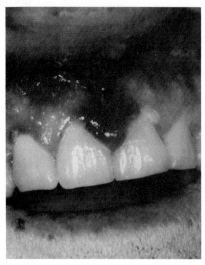

Kaposi's sarcoma

WHITE LESIONS

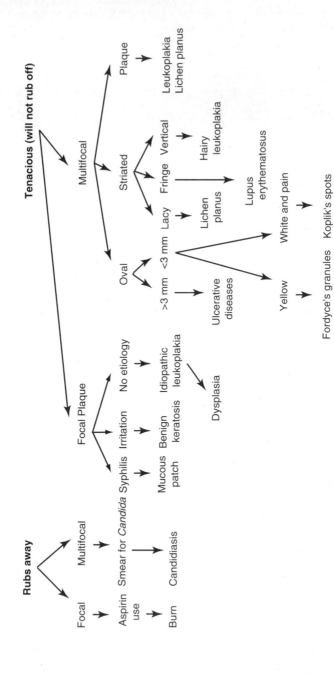

White Lesions

FOCAL PLAQUES

Irritational (frictional) keratosis
Leukoplakia without atypia
Leukoplakia with dysplasia

Significant Findings

1. If the cause is irritation, the primary sources are rubbing dental prostheses and biting of the cheek or lip. The white plaque therefore is localized to the zone of irritation.
2. Leukoplakias do not rub away and are often focal with well-demarcated boundaries. Although both benign and premalignant types are usually seen in tobacco users, leukoplakias also occur in patients who do not use tobacco.

Diagnostic Procedures

1. If a suspected irritant can be identified, it should be eliminated if at all possible. Irritational keratosis can require 1 to 2 months for the mucosa to return to normal. Failure to do so mandates biopsy.
2. All focal white lesions without an irritant source and those associated with smoking or smokeless tobacco should undergo biopsy.

Management

1. Friction- or irritation-induced keratoses are not at great risk for dysplastic change and should be followed and observed. If they fail to resolve within 1 to 2 months following removal of the irritant, they should be assessed microscopically.
2. Benign leukoplakias (those without microscopic evidence of dysplasia) should be followed and observed. Any change in size, configuration, or appearance of either redness or ulceration warrants a second biopsy to determine whether atypical cell changes have evolved with time.
3. Dysplastic leukoplakias must be excised in their entirety by surgery or laser.

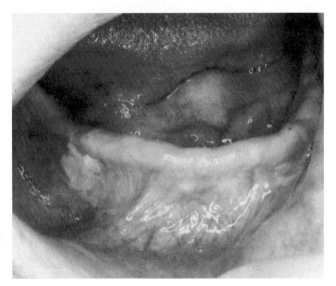

Denture-induced keratosis of the vestibule

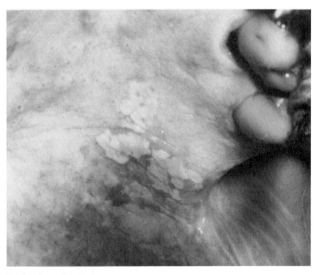

Benign hyperkeratosis

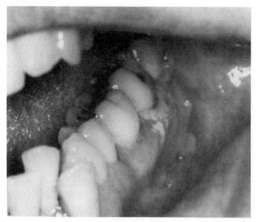

Hyperkeratosis with dysplasia

DIFFUSE BILATERAL WHITE LESIONS

Leukoedema
White sponge nevus
Lichen planus
Leukoplakia

Significant Findings

1. When the white lesions are confined to the buccal mucosa in a dark-skinned patient and the whiteness lessens or disappears after stretching the cheek, leukoedema is the diagnosis.
2. If the lesions are thick, cover the entire buccal mucosa, and occur on the lateral and ventral tongue, and if other family members have similar lesions, the genetically transmitted genokeratosis known as white sponge nevus is most likely.
3. When lesions are in the buccal mucosa and mandibular vestibule, show jagged margins, or exhibit a discrete lacy or spiderweb-like configuration, lichen planus is the probable lesion. One caveat: lupus erythematosus may have a similar appearance.
4. In patients who use smokeless tobacco or who smoke cigarettes, cigars, or a pipe, the lesions probably represent leukoplakias.

Diagnostic Procedures

1. Biopsy is recommended for all diffuse bilateral white lesions except classic leukoedema.
2. Other family members should be examined if white sponge nevus is a consideration.

Management

1. No treatment is needed for leukoedema, white sponge nevus, or benign keratosis.
2. Benign keratosis should be observed and undergo a second biopsy periodically, especially in patients who use tobacco and for lesions that show clinical evidence of change or enlargement. Of particular concern is later malignant transformation, which occurs in 6% of benign leukoplakias. The most ominous changes are ulceration and concomitant erythematous foci (i.e., speckled erythroleukoplakia).
3. Leukoplakia with dysplasia must be excised in its entirety by surgery or laser therapy.

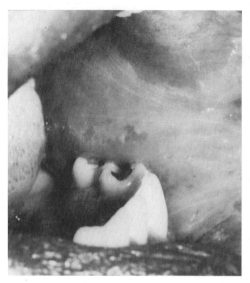

Leukoedema

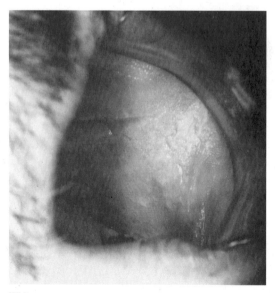

White sponge nevus

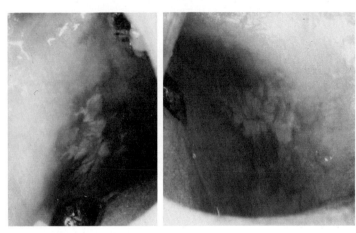

Bilateral lichen planus

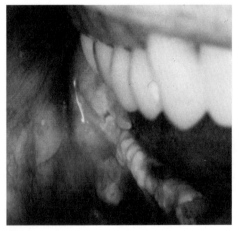

Leukoplakia

MULTIFOCAL PAPULAR WHITE LESIONS

Fordyce's granules
Pseudomembranous candidiasis
Lichen planus
Koplick's spots
Mucous patches (secondary syphilis)

Significant Findings

1. Small (less than 5 mm in diameter), symmetric, yellowish bilateral papules are Fordyce's granules.
2. If the papules have the appearance of curdled milk and rub away, leaving an erythematous base, candidiasis is most likely. Underlying predisposing factors—including diabetes, recent or current antibiotic use, organ transplantation with drug-induced immunosuppression, and HIV infection—should be considered.
3. Papular lesions accompanied by plaques and striae suggest lichen planus.
4. Tiny white papules of the buccal mucosa may represent Koplick's spots, a prodrome of measles. Tincture of time may be required to arrive at a definitive diagnosis.
5. White papules of the lips and buccal mucosa exceeding 5 mm may represent mucous patches. A history of chancre 3 to 6 months previously, either genital or oral, should suggest syphilis.

Diagnostic Procedures

1. A cytologic smear for *Candida* mycelia is necessary in suspected candidiasis.
2. Biopsy may be recommended when a clinical diagnosis cannot be rendered or when lichen planus or mucous patches are suspected. In the latter, spirochete stains may be required.
3. If syphilis is suspected, serologic tests for the disease should be ordered (e.g., VDRL, FTA, TPI).

Management

1. No treatment is necessary for Fordyce's granules, which represent normal oral sebaceous glands.
2. Candidiasis (thrush, pseudomembranous type) can be treated with topical or systemic antifungal agents. Recurrence after treatment is generally indicative of underlying systemic disease, such as immunosuppression, diabetes mellitus, or HIV infection.
3. Syphilis requires systemic oral or intramuscular antibiotic therapy, usually penicillin or a related antibiotic.
4. Measles runs its course in 8 to 12 days and can be treated with antipyretic agents and analgesics (nonsteroidal anti-inflammatory drugs).

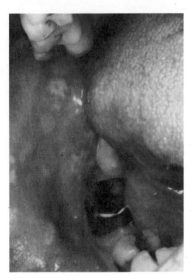

Lichen planus, papular lesions

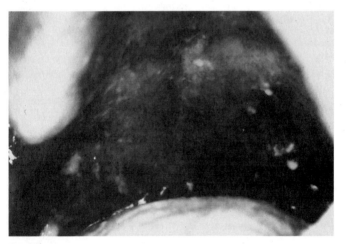

Candidiasis

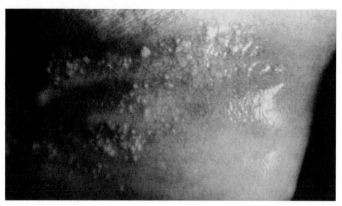

Fordyce's granules

LACE-LIKE AND STRIATED LESIONS

Lichen planus
Hairy leukoplakia
Lupus erythematosus

Significant Findings

1. Lesions are localized to the buccal mucosa and are bilateral in both lichen planus and lupus erythematosus. In lichen planus, the skin lesions are small focal plaques on the wrists and ankles that are pruritic and have a violaceous cast. In lupus erythmatosus, the skin lesions are large and scaly and have a red base. A butterfly rash may be detectable on the face.
2. Vertical striations of the lateral borders of the tongue, usually bilateral, are classic for hairy leukoplakia. This lesion is found in immunocompromised patients, particularly HIV-infected persons.

Diagnostic Procedures

1. Biopsy is necessary for routine pathologic testing, with immunofluorescence and DNA in situ hybridization serving as confirmatory procedures. In lichen planus, basement membrane fibrinogen immunoreactants are seen; in lupus erythematosus, the basement membrane shows a positive lupus band test (i.e., immunoglobulin G or M deposition). DNA probes to Epstein-Barr virus are detected in the epithelium in HIV-infected patients with hairy leukoplakia.
2. Serologic testing for antinuclear antibodies and anti-DNA are positive in lupus erythematosus.

Management

1. Lichen planus requires no treatment unless concomitant erythematous or erosive and ulcerative lesions are present. Topical high-potency steroid gels are then effective.
2. Systemic lupus erythematosus usually requires immunosuppressive drug therapy. Discoid lupus erythematosus with oral lesions, if symptomatic, can be treated with topical steroid gels akin to those used for ulcerative lichen planus.
3. Hairy leukoplakia is asymptomatic and does not require treatment. If patients desire, it can be managed with systemic acyclovir; however, once the medication is withdrawn, the lesions will probably recur.

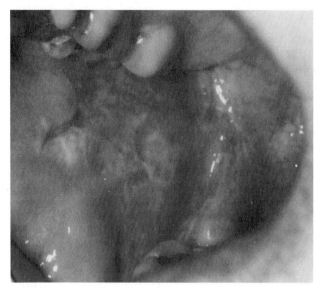

Lichen planus, striae of Wickham

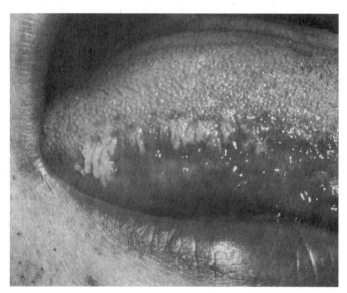

Hairy leukoplakia

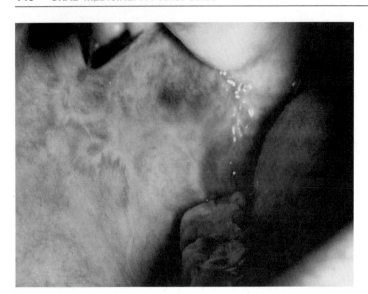

Lupus erythematosus

ULCERATIONS

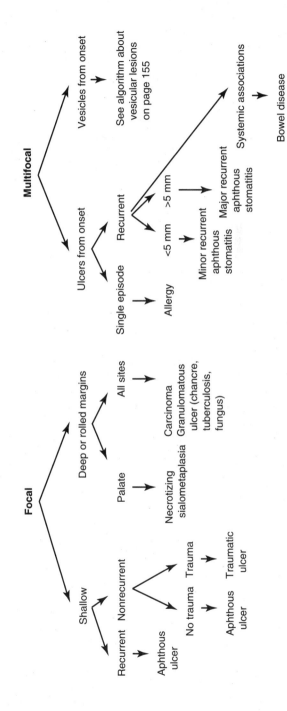

Focal

Shallow
- Recurrent → Aphthous ulcer
- Nonrecurrent
  - No trauma → Aphthous ulcer
  - Trauma → Traumatic ulcer

Deep or rolled margins
- Palate → Necrotizing sialometaplasia
- All sites → Carcinoma
  Granulomatous ulcer (chancre, tuberculosis, fungus)

Multifocal

Vesicles from onset → See algorithm about vesicular lesions on page 155

Ulcers from onset
- Single episode → Allergy
- Recurrent
  - <5 mm → Minor recurrent aphthous stomatitis
  - >5 mm → Major recurrent aphthous stomatitis

Systemic associations →
- Bowel disease
- Gluten enteropathy
- Cyclic neutropenia
- Vitamin B deficiency
- Behçet's syndrome

Ulcerations

SINGLE ULCERS

Traumatic ulcer
Aphthous ulcer
Carcinoma
Granulomatous infection
Necrotizing sialometaplasia

Significant Findings

1. A likely source or history of trauma such as biting or dental appliance irritation can be helpful.
2. A history of recurrences of small round to oval, shallow ulcers is typical of aphthous ulcers.
3. Large ulcers with induration and rolled margins are typical for cancer and granulomatous disease. High-risk sites for cancer are the lateral tongue and floor of the mouth.
4. A history of dyspnea and chronic cough is suggestive of a mycobacterial or mycotic granulomatous infection.
5. Recent (past 2 to 4 weeks) orogenital contact suggests the possibility of syphilitic chancre.
6. A large, deep ulcer at the junction of the hard and soft palates, without rolled margins, suggests necrotizing sialometaplasia.

Diagnostic Procedures

1. Remove any suspected source of trauma or irritation. Traumatic ulcers heal in 10 to 14 days.
2. All ulcers that persist for more than 2 weeks should undergo biopsy, as should deep-seated large ulcers, particularly those with rolled borders.
3. Recurrent aphthous ulceration (stomatitis) can usually be diagnosed by clinical appearance and history of recurrence.

Management

1. Minor recurrent aphthae can be managed by application of topical anti-inflammatory and steroid gel preparations.
2. Biopsy will disclose cancerous change in nonhealing ulcers. Squamous cell carcinoma, salivary adenocarcinomas, and lymphomas can all present with single or focal ulcerations. Referral to the appropriate cancer specialist is required.
3. Granulomatous diseases, with the exception of syphilis, are usually associated with pulmonary infection. Referral to an infectious disease specialist is recommended. Oral chancre that has been confirmed by biopsy and treponemal stains is treated with penicillin-related antibiotics.

4. Once the diagnosis of necrotizing sialometaplasia has been confirmed by biopsy, the ulcer will spontaneously resolve in 2 to 3 weeks.

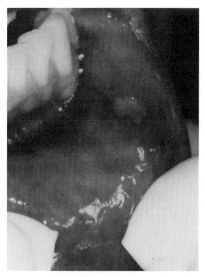

Aphthous ulcer

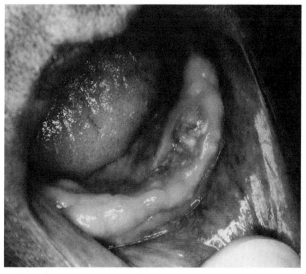

Squamous cell carcinoma

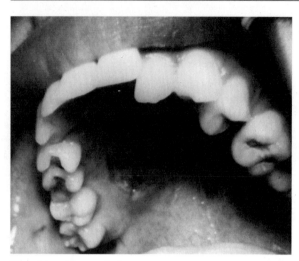

Necrotizing sialometaplasia

MULTIPLE AND RECURRENT ULCERS

Minor aphthae
Major aphthae
Herpetiform aphthae
Viral stomatitis
Allergic stomatitis
Gluten enteropathy
Inflammatory bowel disease
Cyclic neutropenia
Agranulocytosis
Vitamin B complex or folate deficiency
HIV-associated cytomegalovirus
HIV-associated aphthous-like ulcer

Significant Findings

1. Assessment of size and configuration is significant. Small oval ulcers represent minor aphthae, whereas ulcers more than 5 mm in diameter in conjunction with scarring are more likely to represent major aphthae. Herpetiform ulcers are the smallest (2 to 4 mm) and are plentiful (20 to 30 lesions each episode). Agranulocytic and cyclic neutropenia ulcers are usually large, shallow, and of irregular outline.
2. A history of recurrence is indicative of an aphtha or a viral ulceration.
3. Movable mucosa is typical for aphthae; fixed mucosa is typical for viral (herpetic) ulcers, which are most often seen on the palatal gingiva adjacent to the premolar and first molar teeth.
4. Viral vesiculoulcerative lesions cluster together in groups, since recurrent herpes exits multiple individual axons from a given nerve.
5. When vesicles precede the ulcer, it is of viral origin.
6. Underlying systemic illness may be present. Aphthous-like ulcerations occur in vitamin B deficiencies, gluten enteropathy, chronic inflammatory bowel diseases, agranulocytosis from cancer chemotherapy, and HIV infection.
7. Frequent upper respiratory infections and advanced periodontal disease in adolescents suggest cyclic neutropenia, a rare blood dyscrasia.

Diagnostic Procedures

1. When bowel symptoms are extant (e.g., abdominal pain, chronic and intermittent diarrhea or constipation, buoyant stools), a diagnostic workup for intestinal disease should be undertaken. Gastrointestinal imaging series and assessment for gliadin allergy are to be included.

2. Hemogram is required for suspected agranulocytic ulcers. When cyclic neutropenia is suspected, weekly white and differential blood cell counts should be obtained over a 5-week period.
3. Biopsy is indicated only in large ulcers, particularly those occurring in HIV-infected patients, in whom virus (herpes simplex virus, cytomegalovirus) may be causative. Specific immunostains or in situ hybridization may be useful.
4. Referral to an allergist for immediate type I hypersensitivity assessment is in order if a food or drug allergy is suspected.

Management

1. Aphthae are treated by topical corticosteroids, tetracycline rinses, or, in severe or major episodes (including HIV-associated ulcers), systemic pulse prednisone.
2. Recurrent ulcers related to systemic diseases—including bowel disease, gluten enteropathy, and neutropenia—resolve when appropriate therapy is instituted for the medical condition. Palliation can be attained with analgesic or antihistaminic mouth rinses in conjunction with topical corticosteroids.
3. Cytomegalovirus ulcers in HIV are generally associated with more widespread infection (pulmonary, ocular). Gancyclovir therapy is usually instituted.
4. Documented allergic reactions are treated by withdrawal of allergen and administration of systemic antihistamines (immediate), steroids (contact or erythema multiforme-like ulcerations), or both.

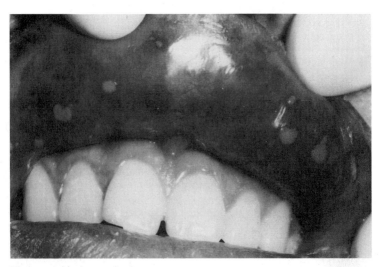

Viral stomatitis, herpes simplex

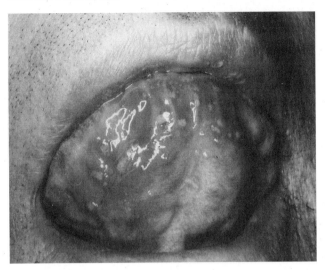

Allergic stomatitis

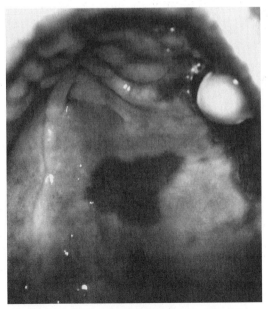

Agranulocytic ulcers in patient taking anticancer medication

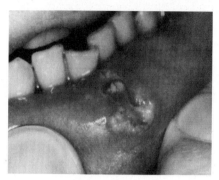

Cytomegalovirus ulcer in HIV-positive patient

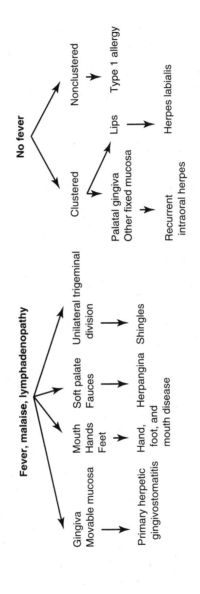

VESICULAR LESIONS

Fever, malaise, lymphadenopathy

Gingiva Movable mucosa	Mouth Hands Feet	Soft palate Fauces	Unilateral trigeminal division
↓	↓	↓	↓
Primary herpetic gingivostomatitis	Hand, foot, and mouth disease	Herpangina	Shingles

No fever

Clustered

Palatal gingiva / Other fixed mucosa → Recurrent intraoral herpes

Lips → Herpes labialis

Nonclustered → Type 1 allergy

Vesicular Eruptions

Herpes simplex
    Primary herpetic gingivostomatitis
    Recurrent herpes labialis
    Recurrent intraoral herpes
Varicella zoster
    Chickenpox
    Shingles
Coxsackievirus
    Herpangina
    Hand, foot, and mouth disease
Allergic stomatitis

Significant Findings

1. If the lesions appear as punctuate ulcers, it is important to verify that they began as vesicles. If they began, from their inception, as ulcers, see Multiple and Recurrent Ulcerations.
2. If the patient is febrile, primary viral infection is the probable cause. If not, secondary or recurrent viral infection or allergy is likely.
3. A history of previous episodes or clustering into a focal group indicates herpes simplex.
4. When the vesicles follow the nerve supply, stopping abruptly at the midline, shingles is probable.
5. Concurrent skin lesions are present in shingles and hand, foot, and mouth disease.
6. Localization:
   a. Lips or unilateral hard palate—recurrent herpes simplex
   b. Attached gingiva and movable mucosa—primary herpes simplex
   c. Soft palate—herpangina
   d. Mouth, hands, feet—hand, foot, and mouth disease
7. When lesions persist for more than 1 month, underlying HIV disease should be suspected.
8. Consumption of any "new" foods, use of a new brand of mouth rinse, or history of taking any medication just before the onset of a vesicular eruption suggests IgE-mediated hypersensitivity.

Diagnostic Procedures

1. Clinical findings and localization of vesicles usually establish the diagnosis.
2. Smear of an intact vesicle or vesicular fluids is required to uncover herpes-specific cytologic evidence of keratinocyte ballooning degeneration.
3. Smear for viral antigen-specific immunoperoxidase or DNA in situ hybridization is recommended.

4. Stool culture for coxsackievirus is recommended.
5. Specific serum titers, active and convalescent, should be assessed.

Management

1. Palliative mouth rinses (antihistamines, anesthetics) are helpful.
2. Herpes group viruses (herpes simplex, varicella zoster) can be treated with topical and systemic acyclovir.
3. Specific antivirals are not available for coxsackieviruses.
4. Allergic stomatitis is treated with systemic antihistamines.

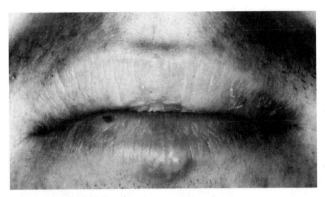

Recurrent herpes labialis

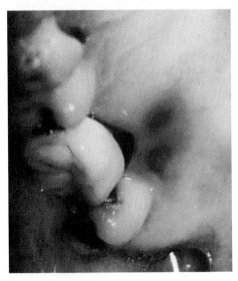

Recurrent intraoral herpes

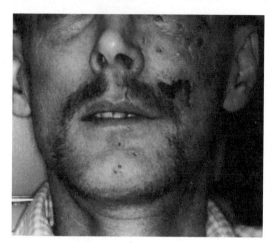

Second division zoster

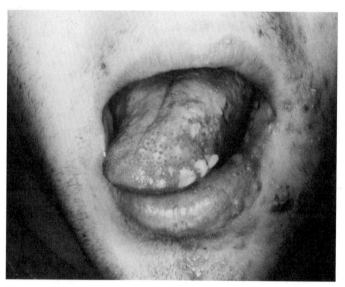

Third division zoster

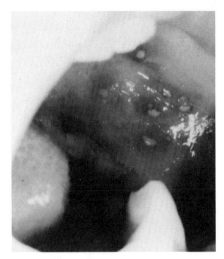

Coxsackievirus stomatitis

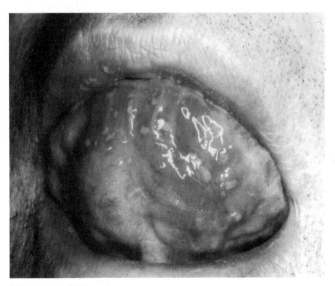

Allergy to shellfish

BULLOUS–DESQUAMATIVE LESIONS

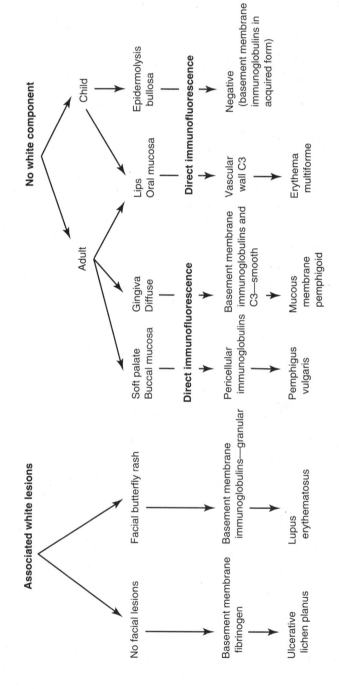

Bullous–Desquamative Lesions

Erosive lichen planus
Mucous membrane pemphigoid
Bullous pemphigoid
Pemphigus vulgaris
Erythema multiforme
    Minor
    Major (Stevens-Johnson syndrome)
Epidermolysis bullosa

Significant Findings

1. When white striae are apparent or when lesions are bilateral in the vestibule and buccal mucosa, lichen planus is most likely.
2. If lesions are localized primarily on the facial gingiva, mucous membrane pemphigoid is most likely.
3. When the lesions are located primarily on the soft palate, pemphigus vulgaris is probable.
4. Extensive crusting lesions of the lips are typical for erythema multiforme.
5. All bullous diseases may show skin bullae, except mucous membrane pemphigoid, in which skin lesions are rare. Target lesions are erythema multiforme; target lesions in combination with ocular and genital erosions indicate Stevens-Johnson syndrome (erythema multiforme major).
6. A history of recent drug intake, particularly sulfas, is indicative of erythema multiforme.
7. A precedent herpes virus infection also suggests immune complex erythema multiforme.
8. Most bullous–desquamative lesions occur in adults, except for epidermolysis bullosa, a group of bullous diseases arising in childhood or infancy.
9. Mucosal Nikolsky's sign can be seen in all of the bullous lesions; it is not diagnostic for pemphigus.

Diagnostic Procedures

1. Cytologic smear is useful only in pemphigus vulgaris to show Tzanck cells.
2. Biopsy usually provides for a definitive diagnosis:
   a. Bandlike lymphocytic infiltrate with basal cell lysis indicates erosive lichen planus.
   b. Subbasilar split is a sign of bullous pemphigoid or mucous membrane pemphigoid.
   c. Suprabasilar split indicates pemphigus vulgaris.
3. Direct immunofluorescence:
   a. Anti–basement membrane IgG, IgM, or C3 occurs in mucous membrane pemphigoid, bullous pemphigoid, and lupus erythematosus.

   b. Anti–basement membrane IgA typifies linear IgA disease.
   c. Anti–intercellular cement IgG, IgM, or C3 indicates pemphigus vulgaris.
   d. Perivascular IgG, IgM, or C3 is seen in erythema multiforme.
   e. Anti–basement membrane fibrinogen indicates lichen planus.

Management

1. Topical corticosteroids and steroid mouth rinses are used for local control; cyclosporine rinses are efficacious for lichen planus as well.
2. Systemic prednisone is required for severe involvement.
3. Dapsone is used for bullous pemphigoid or mucous membrane pemphigoid.
4. Azathioprine with prednisone is necessary for steroid-refractory cases.

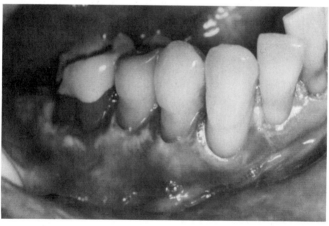

Erosive lichen planus

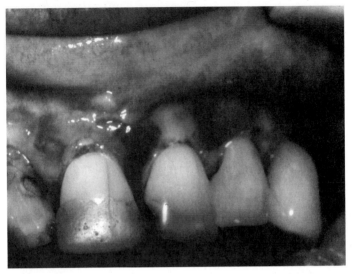

Mucous membrane pemphigoid

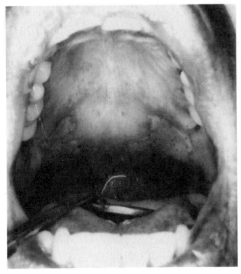

Pemphigus vulgaris

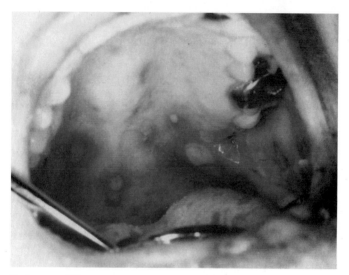

Erythema multiforme

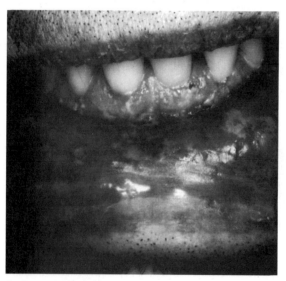

Erythema multiforme

FOCAL PIGMENTED LESIONS

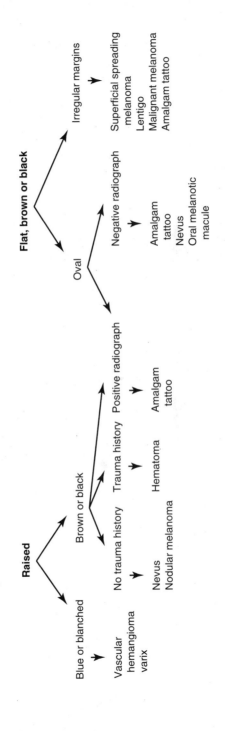

MULTIFOCAL PIGMENTED LESIONS

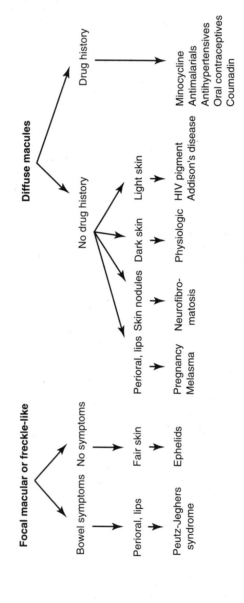

Pigmented Lesions

FOCAL GRAY, BLACK, AND BROWN MACULES

Amalgam tattoo
Graphite tattoo
Focal melanotic macule (ephelis)
Junctional nevus
Blue nevus
Ecchymosis
Superficial spreading melanoma

Significant Findings

1. Amalgam tattoo is most common; melanoma least likely.
2. History:
    a. Sudden onset—melanoma likely
    b. Present many years, no change—benign condition
    c. Recent bite or injury—ecchymosis probable
3. Location:
    a. Adjacent to a large restoration or crown—tattoo
    b. Hard palate—probable graphite tattoo
    c. Lower lip—probable ephelis
    d. Anterior maxillary gingiva—melanoma probable
4. Radiographic evidence of opaque particles is indicative of a tattoo.

Diagnostic Procedures

1. If opaque particles are evident on a radiograph, a tattoo is likely and the patient can be placed on clinical follow-up.
2. If no metal particles are seen, biopsy should be considered.
3. If there is sudden onset with no trauma history, biopsy is indicated.

Management

1. Lesions suspected to represent amalgam tattoos, the most common of oral focal pigmentations, should be followed to ensure that no changes occur; an increase in size indicates the probability of another type of lesion.
2. When biopsy discloses any of the above-listed diagnoses other than melanoma, no further treatment is necessary.
3. When the diagnosis is hematoma or ecchymosis, a bleeding disorder should be considered, especially if excessive or poorly controlled bleeding occurs during biopsy or when other ecchymotic areas appear without provocation. Prothrombin time, partial thromboplastin time, complete blood count, platelet count, and bleeding time should be obtained.

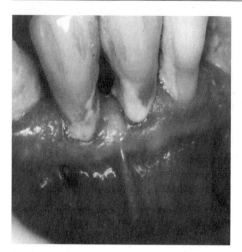

Amalgam tattoo

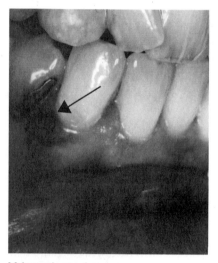

Melanocytic macule

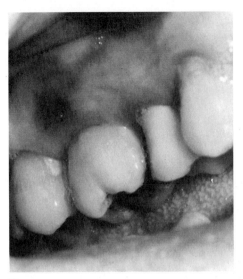

Nevus

MULTIPLE GRAY, BLACK, AND BROWN MACULES

Multiple amalgam tattoos
Physiologic (ethnic) pigmentation
Peutz-Jeghers syndrome
von Recklinghausen neurofibromatosis
Albright's syndrome
Cushing's syndrome
Addison's disease
Drug-induced hyperpigmentation
Smoker's melanosis
Chloasma (melasma)
HIV-associated oral melanosis

Significant Findings

1. Common lesions include multiple amalgam tattoos, physiologic (ethnic) pigmentation, and smoker's melanosis. The rest are rare.
2. The presence of large restorations adjacent to lesions or radiographic evidence of opaque particles indicates amalgam tattoos.
3. Perioral locations, macules on fingers, and gastrointestinal complaints are indicative of Peutz-Jeghers syndrome with intestinal polyposis.
4. Dark skin, hair, eyes, and oral mucosa are from physiologic (ethnic) pigmentation.
5. Long history of smoking predisposes for smoker's melanosis.
6. For bronzing of the skin without sun exposure but with accompanying hypotension or hypoglycemia, a workup for adrenal hypocorticism is necessary.
7. For bronzing of the skin without sun exposure but with accompanying hypertension or hyperglycemia, a workup for ACTH-secreting neoplasm (nonadrenal Cushing's syndrome) with secondary hypercorticism is necessary.
8. If the patient is HIV-seropositive, HIV oral melanosis is a possibility, or it may be due to opportunistic infection involving adrenal cortex with secondary Addison's disease, even in patients with HIV infection.
9. Long-term antibiotic therapy minocycline can cause drug-induced melanosis.
10. If the patient is pregnant or taking birth control pills, melasma or chloasma is likely.
11. Cutaneous café-au-lait macules with multiple nodules or pendulous tumors indicate neurofibromatosis.
12. Osseous lesions, deformities or fractures, precocious puberty, thyroid enlargement, and cutaneous pigmentation are signs of polyostotic fibrous dysplasia with endocrinopathy (Albright's syndrome).

Diagnostic Procedures

1. Most of these diseases show microscopic evidence of basilar melanosis with some degree of melanin incontinence. Therefore, biopsy is not particularly helpful other than to confirm the benign nature of the disease.
2. Many diffuse and multifocal oral pigmented macules are associated with specific accompaniments. The diagnosis is based on association with other specific findings. Cutaneous, osseous, and intestinal complaints or lesions should be sought and endocrinopathic disease considered, with emphasis placed on procuring a thorough medical history.
3. Pregnancy and drug intake, including birth control pills and specific antibiotics, should be considered in the pathogenesis.
4. Physical diagnosis and laboratory tests may be in order. In Addison's disease and Cushing's syndrome, blood pressure and serum glucose are altered. HIV-associated pigmentation may be accompanied by other physical signs, such as oral candidiasis, hairy leukoplakia, or Kaposi's sarcoma, and HIV serologic testing may be in order.

Management

1. No treatment or management is needed for the following:
   a. Documented amalgam tattoos
   b. Physiologic (ethnic) melanosis
   c. Smoker's melanosis—Consider smoking cessation program.
   d. HIV melanosis—If other diagnostic possibilities are not uncovered and HIV risk factors are present or suspected, HIV testing should be considered.
   e. Chloasma—Consider cessation of birth control pills, with institution of alternative birth control methods. Pregnancy-associated pigmentation usually resolves after parturition.
2. Addison's disease (adrenal hypocorticism) requires complete medical workup and treatment of the underlying cause (e.g., granulomatous disease, autoimmune cortical destruction).
3. Cushing's syndrome with secondary hypercorticism is due to a pituitary lesion or a steroid- or ACTH-secreting carcinoma (e.g., small cell carcinoma of the lung).
4. Albright's and von Recklinghausen's syndromes should be managed by orthopaedists and dermatologists, respectively. There is no curative treatment available for either of these rare diseases.
5. Perioral macular pigmentation should arouse suspicion of intestinal polyposis, and referral to a gastroenterologist is recommended.

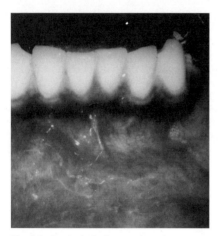

Physiologic gingival pigmentation

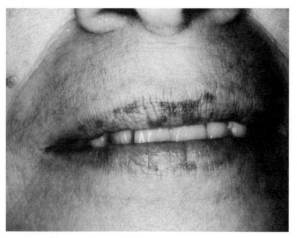

Peutz-Jeghers syndrome

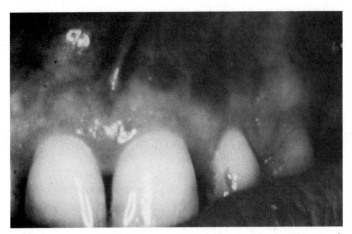

Gingival pigment in HIV infection

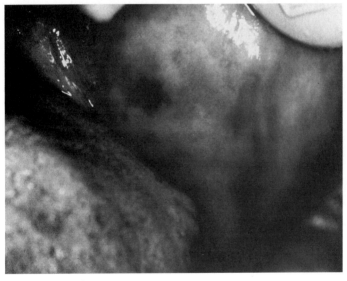

Smoker's melanosis

RED LESIONS*

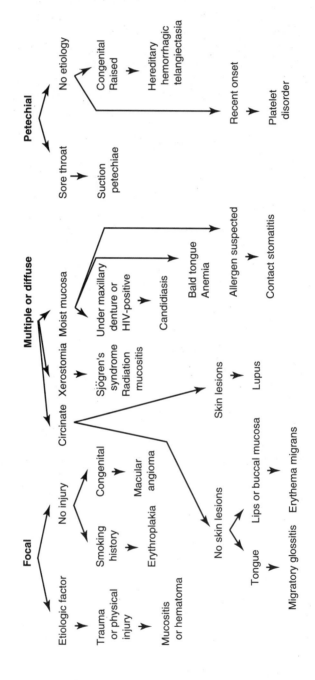

*If ulceration, desquamation, or bullous lesions are evident, see other appropriate algorithms.

Red Lesions

Petechiae

Suction petechiae
Thrombocytopenic purpura
Thrombocytopathia
Leukemia
Hereditary hemorrhagic telangiectasia

Significant Findings

1. Localization to soft palate usually indicates suction petechiae.
2. History of sore, itchy throat, malaise, and fever with lymphade-nopathy suggests infectious mononucleosis, cold, or flu. Patients tend to click the itchy soft palate with the posterior aspect of the tongue.
3. Presence of cutaneous as well as mucosal lesions is indicative of a blood dyscrasia.
4. Malaise and gingival enlargement with generalized pallor suggest leukemia.
5. Drug history (e.g., anticancer medications, which induce bone marrow suppression, or aspirin, which inhibits platelet aggrega-tion) may cause petechiae.
6. Familial history, slightly papular appearance, and involvement of the nasal mucosa are indicative of hereditary hemorrhagic telangiectasia.

Diagnostic Procedures

1. Bleeding time is prolonged when platelet disorders are present.
2. A complete blood count with differential is necessary to test for leukemia.
3. Platelet count is necessary to determine the presence of thrombo-cytopenia. Further evaluation for etiology includes leukemia workup, drug history, autoimmune platelet lysis, HIV-associated idiopathic thrombocytopenic purpura.
4. Platelet aggregation assays can detect drug-induced and genetic defects in platelet aggregation proteins (e.g., aspirin-induced cyclo-oxygenase inhibition in platelet thromboxane production or von Willebrand factor VIII adhesion protein).
5. HIV testing should be conducted when risk factors are evident or other lesions suggestive of HIV disease coexist with the petechial lesions.
6. Monospot testing is necessary for suspected mononucleosis.
7. In suspected hereditary hemorrhagic telangiectasia, a punch biopsy can be revealing.

Management

1. When a blood dyscrasia is uncovered, refer the patient to the appropriate specialist (e.g., hematologist, oncologist).

2. *Do not* render any oral surgical care until the basis for the hemorrhagic diathesis is uncovered. Platelet counts under 50,000 will result in uncontrollable hemorrhage. Aggregation below 50% of normal will result in prolonged bleeding. Emergency dental surgery should be done in the hospital, where platelet infusions are available.
3. Suction petechiae of the soft palate due to fellatio or clicking of an itchy palate resolve in 2 to 3 days.
4. Mononucleosis is treated by bed rest and analgesics.
5. No treatment is necessary for hereditary hemorrhagic telangiectasia. Epistaxis can be a problem.

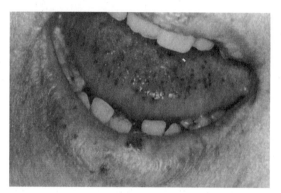

Hereditary hemorrhagic telangiectasia

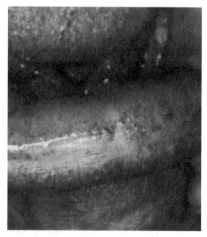

Lip petechiae in thrombocytopenia

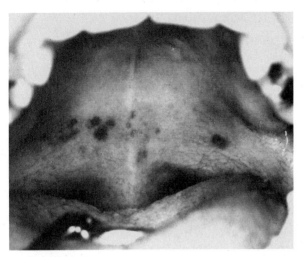

Suction petechiae

FOCAL ERYTHEMATOUS MACULES

Nonspecific mucositis
Macular hemangioma
Ecchymosis
Erythroplakia

Significant Findings

1. Search out an etiologic factor. Most focal red lesions are inflammatory lesions secondary to injury or a thermal burn to the mucosa. Alternatively, recent trauma may have caused localized extravasation of blood or ecchymosis. Such lesions should resolve in 7 to 10 days.
2. Duration is important, since macular hemangiomas are generally congenital or evolve during childhood years.
3. A history of smoking and heavy alcohol use should arouse suspicion of a precancerous erythroplakia. Some lesions are speckled with white foci, representing either superimposed candidiasis or foci of keratosis.

Diagnostic Procedures

1. Suspected reactions to injury should be confirmed by history or examination (e.g., pizza burn, cheek biting, tongue biting, iatrogenic injuries). Such lesions should be observed at 10 days for resolution.
2. If no cancer risk factors are present and the patient has had the lesion for many years, an attempt should be made to compress the lesion to check for blanching. If the macule blanches under pressure, a clinical diagnosis of macular hemangioma can be made and the lesion can then be followed to make sure no increase in size occurs. Most mucosal macular angiomas are a component of facial skin port-wine hemangiomas. A diagnosis of Sturge-Weber syndrome is made only when intracranial angiomas are extant and there is a history of seizures.
3. Biopsy is recommended, particularly in patients who smoke and drink heavily. Precancerous erythroplakia is the chief consideration.

Management

1. Nonspecific mucositis due to injury will resolve in 7 to 10 days after the etiologic agent has been eliminated.
2. Angiomas are usually left untreated.
3. Erythroplakias with dysplasia or carcinoma in situ can be treated by surgical or laser excision or by radiation therapy. Invasive carcinoma arising in erythroplakia has metastatic potential and should be treated more aggressively.

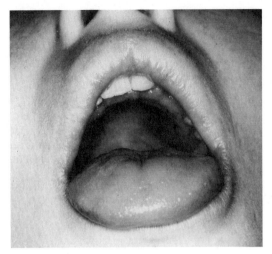

Palatal nonspecific mucositis secondary to use of an orthodontic appliance

MULTIPLE, CIRCINATE, DISCOID LESIONS

Benign migratory glossitis
Erythema areata migrans
Lupus erythematosus

Significant Findings

1. Localization to the tongue with no symptoms or only minor discomfort and depapillated foci with a circinate hypertrophic white marginal rim is typical for migratory glossitis. A history of clearing with relocation is classic.
2. Mucosal localization with red oval foci in the absence of significant pain or burning symptoms, a circinate whitish rim, and a history of clearing and reappearance at a new site are typical for erythema migrans.
3. Concomitant skin lesions, especially a butterfly rash of the face or scaly erythematous skin plaques, are suggestive of lupus.

Diagnostic Procedures

1. The clinical features of migratory glossitis and erythema migrans are usually pathognomonic. One important caveat is to recall that dysplastic lesions can be red (erythroplakia). Biopsy is therefore recommended when a solitary lesion is present and when there is a history of smoking or alcohol abuse.
2. Suspected cases of lupus should undergo biopsy with immunofluorescence testing to uncover basement membrane–bound immunoglobulins (lupus band test). Serologic testing for antinuclear antibodies and anti-DNA autoantibodies is also recommended. Recall that lupus erythematosus can be cutaneous (discoid) or systemic with significant renal involvement. Young females are most often affected.

Management

1. The causes of migratory glossitis and erythema areata migrans are unknown. No treatment is needed. Some patients, however, complain of mild burning, which can be managed with an antihistaminic mouth rinse.
2. A diagnosis of lupus erythematosus requires medical consultation. Immunosuppressive agents may be needed; in such instances, resolution of the oral lesions may occur. Discoid lupus erythematosus with oral lesions can be managed by topical high-potency corticosteroid gels.

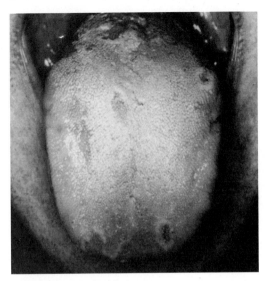

Benign migratory glossitis

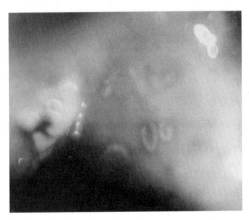

Erythema areata migrans

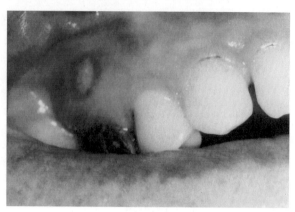

Lupus erythematosus

DIFFUSE HOMOGENEOUS ERYTHEMAS

Erythematous candidiasis and denture sore mouth
Bald tongue–associated anemias
Sjögren's syndrome
Contact stomatitis

Significant Findings

1. Depapillation of the tongue, in the absence of lesions elsewhere on the mucosa, is suggestive of pernicious anemia or folate deficiency.
2. If dryness is a complaint, other features of either primary or secondary Sjögren's syndrome should be sought (e.g., parotid enlargement, xerophthalmia, lupoid skin lesions, joint pain, and swelling).
3. Confinement of red lesions to the denture-bearing zone of the hard palate is most suggestive of denture sore mouth with associated erythematous candidiasis.
4. Question the patient about any putative contact allergens that may have coincided with onset of oral symptoms. Chief considerations include new dentifrices, mouth rinses, and foods.
5. Recent antibiotic use or underlying systemic diseases—including HIV infection, diabetes, cancer, and cancer chemotherapy—are often associated with candidiasis, either pseudomembranous or erythematous.

Diagnostic Procedures

1. When xerostomia is present, serologic tests should be conducted for autoimmune sialadenitis and for collagen diseases, including tests for rheumatoid factor, antinuclear antibodies, anti-Rho, and anti-La. A lower lip biopsy for lymphocyte focus score is also recommended.
2. A hemogram is in order for suspected anemia. This can be performed in conjunction with measurements of serum folate and vitamin B_{12} levels, along with gastric analysis for achlorhydria.
3. Cytologic smear is necessary for identification of *Candida* mycelia (they are not always evident in the erythematous form of candidiasis). Serum glucose and HIV testing can be considered in patients suspected to be at risk for diabetes and AIDS, respectively.
4. Withdrawal of any suspected allergenic substances is appropriate, with subsequent rechallenge to document a cause-and-effect relationship.

Management

1. Sjögren's syndrome management requires palliative mouth rinses and saliva substitutes, as well as daily topical fluoride gels for caries prevention.

2. For denture sore mouth, topical cream or gel should be applied to the inner surface of the denture. A soft reline may be in order as well. Diffuse erythematous candidiasis can be treated with systemic or topical antifungal agents.
3. Pernicious anemia requires therapy with injectable vitamin B_{12}. Oral folate can reverse folic acid–deficiency anemia.
4. For contact allergy, topical steroid gels or steroid mouth rinses are necessary, along with removal of the suspected allergen.

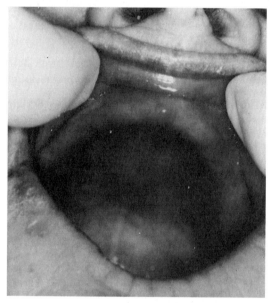

Candidiasis

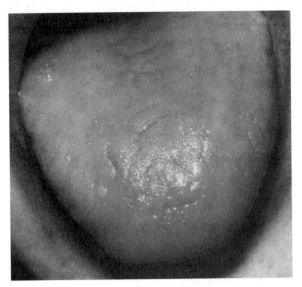

Bald tongue in a patient with pernicious anemia

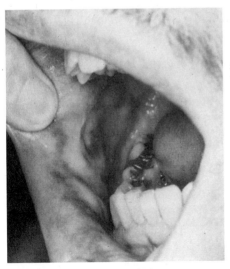

Contact stomatitis reaction to cinnamon

Oral and Maxillofacial Lesions Caused by Medications/Chemicals

Certain prescription and over-the-counter medications can have adverse effects on the tissues of the head and neck region. Ulcerations, desquamations, pigmentations, infections, purpura, soft tissue enlargements, dry mouth, and facial deformities can all be caused by drugs. The medication history is therefore highly relevant to the differential diagnosis of oral and maxillofacial disease, even though medication-related lesions are not as common as disease processes unrelated to drugs. Listed here are the major classes of drugs that have been associated with specific lesions.

MUCOCUTANEOUS AND DENTAL PIGMENTATIONS

Birth control pills—can cause melasma, a diffuse macular melanosis of the perioral and periorbital facial skin

Minocycline—antibiotic associated with mucosal macular diffuse melanosis

Tetracycline—if used by the pregnant mother during fetal tooth development, can cause hard tissue yellow or brown pigmentation that fluoresces green under ultraviolet light

Lead—if ingested (usually while consuming paint), can cause linear pigmentation of the gingiva

Chlorhexidine—can cause brown pigment deposition of the teeth and brown coloration of the dorsal tongue

Griseofulvin—can cause a black coating of the dorsal tongue

ERYTHEMA MULTIFORME

Considered an allergic disease mediated by either IgE or immune complex vasculitis, erythema multiforme is often caused by medications, although postherpetic disease is also a common cause. The list of drugs that can precipitate erythema multiforme is long, so only the more common are tabulated here.

Sulfa antibiotics—used to treat urinary tract infections

Sulfonylurea hypoglycemic agents—used to lower glucose level in non–insulin dependent diabetes

Other antibiotics (chloramphenicol, ciprofloxacin, penicillins, tetracyclines, clindamycin, dapsone, isoniazid, griseofulvin)—used to treat infections

Anticonvulsants (carbamazepine, phenytoin)—used to treat epilepsy and trigeminal neuralgia

Analgesics (aspirin, barbiturates, codeine, nonsteroidal antiinflammatory drugs)—employed in inflammatory conditions

Antihypertensives (diltiazem, hydralazine, verapamil, minoxidil)—for blood pressure diminution

Psychotherapeutics (glutethimide, lithium, meprobamate)—for personality disorders

Cimetidine—used to treat peptic/gastric ulcers

PURPURA (PETECHIAE, ECCHYMOSES)

Anticancer chemotherapeutic agents (e.g., cyclophosphamide, 5-fluorouracil, methotrexate, mitomycin, bleomycin, doxorubicin, vinblastine)—can cause bone marrow suppression and thrombocytopenia

Antihypertensive agents, ACE inhibitors, and beta-blockers—can cause myelosuppression with thrombocytopenia

CANDIDIASIS

Antibiotics (various) —allow overgrowth of the fungal flora in *Candida* carriers

Systemic steroids—used to manage collagen/immune diseases on a long-term basis; confer susceptibility to candidiasis.

VESICULOULCERATIVE LESIONS

Immunosuppressive drugs (steroids, azathioprine)—predispose to herpesvirus infections; used to manage organ transplantation and collagen/immune diseases

Anticancer chemotherapeutic agents (e.g., cyclophosphamide, 5-fluorouracil, methotrexate, mitomycin, bleomycin, doxorubicin, vinblastine)—can cause bone marrow suppression and neutropenia

Antihypertensives, ACE inhibitors, beta-blockers—can cause myelosuppression with neutropenia

Antibiotics (penicillin, erythromycin)—can cause type 1 hypersensitivity manifested as vesiculoulcerative stomatitis

Dental resin monomer—can cause type 4 contact hypersensitivity stomatitis

Antioxidants (octyl gallate)—used as a preservative in lip balms, lipsticks, and foods; can cause allergic ulcerations

PEMPHIGUS VULGARIS

Penicillamine—used in the treatment of Wilson's disease; can stimulate a reversible production of pemphigus autoantibodies

Angiotensin-converting enzyme antihypertensives (captopril)—can stimulate a reversible production of pemphigus autoantibodies

LICHENOID REACTIONS AND KERATOSES

Gold salts—used to treat arthritis and multiple sclerosis
Dental metals (particularly mercury and nickel in amalgams, orthodontic brackets, and wires)—direct mucosal contact allergy
Dental resins—direct mucosal contact allergy
Cinnaminic aldehyde—direct mucosal contact of foods or chewing gum containing cinnamon flavoring elicits T-cell response in some patients
Quinidine (antimalarial agent)
Photographic processing chemicals—topical lichenoid reactions
Alcoholic mouthwashes—can induce diffuse white lesions with excessive use
Dentifrices, anti-tartar agents—can cause white lesions with superficial desquamation

LUPUS-LIKE DRUG REACTIONS

Many drugs have been reported to cause lupus erythematosus–like disease. Only those drugs with a well-documented association are listed here.
Chlorpromazine—anxiolytic and antiemetic agent
Hydralazine—antihypertensive, direct-acting vasodilator
Isoniazid—antibiotic against tuberculosis
Alpha-methyldopa—central-acting antihypertensive agent
Procainamide—antiarrhythmic agent

GINGIVAL HYPERPLASIA

Cyclosporine—immunosuppressive drug used in patients undergoing organ transplantation
Dilantin (hydantoin)—antiseizure medication
Calcium channel blockers (particularly nifedipine)—vascular wall–stabilizing drugs used to treat angina and hypertension

ANGIOEDEMA

Facial swelling from IgE or IgG/complement-mediated allergy is referred to as angioedema. Skin urticaria is often seen as well.
Angiotensin-converting enzyme antihypertensive agents (captopril)
Other antihypertensive agents (beta-blockers, diuretics)
Antibiotics (penicillin, cephalosporin, sulfa drugs)
Nonsteroidal anti-inflammatory drugs
Vaccines
Opiates
Sedatives, anxiolytic agents
Doxorubicin

FACIAL DEFORMITIES AND CLEFTS
(IN UTERO TERATOGENS)

Systemic corticosteroids—if taken during first trimester of pregnancy

XEROSTOMIA

Numerous medications have an anticholinergic effect on the salivary glands. Below is a partial listing of the drugs that most often cause dry mouth.
Tricyclic and tetracyclic antidepressants
Anticholinergic agents
Diuretics
Antihistamines
Antihypertensives
Nonsteroidal anti-inflammatory agents
Antipsychotic agents
Anorexic drugs and amphetamines
Anxiolytic agents
Antiparkinsonian agents
Laxatives
Antiulcer medications
Various combination nonprescription drugs—used to treat cold, influenza, and allergy symptoms

Oral and Maxillofacial Lesions Associated With Systemic Disease

Oral, jaw, and facial skin lesions are usually entities unto themselves; however, many systemic diseases have oral and maxillofacial manifestations. The lesions that occur in conjunction with or as a component of systemic diseases are listed according to clinical appearance.

MUCOCUTANEOUS PIGMENTATIONS

Pregnancy—Some patients develop malasma, a diffuse macular melanosis of the perioral and periorbital facial skin.
Neurofibromatosis (von Recklinghausen's disease of skin)—This heritable disease is characterized by multiple skin nodules or pendulous tumors and brown macular pigmentations that may involve the head and neck skin. Intraoral café-au-lait pigmentation is rare.
Fibrous dysplasia—Albright's syndrome, which is characterized by polyostotic fibrous dysplasia, precocious puberty, thyroid enlargement, and café-au-lait pigmentation of the skin and mucosa, is extremely rare.

Pituitary-based adrenal hypercorticism (Cushing's syndrome)—ACTH hypersecretion from the posterior pituitary results in a secondary adrenocortical hyperplasia. The elevated ACTH has melanocyte-stimulating effects, and both oral and facial pigmentation may be seen. Nonpituitary, neuroendocrine carcinomas can also secrete ACTH.

Adrenal insufficiency (Addison's disease)—Depressed steroid production feeds back to the pituitary, with elevation in ACTH levels. The elevated ACTH has melanocyte-stimulating effects, and both oral and facial pigmentation may be seen.

Peutz-Jeghers syndrome—In this hereditary disease characterized by intestinal polyposis without a significant predisposition to carcinomatous transformation, multiple perioral and digital macular, freckle-like pigmentations are classically encountered.

HIV-associated pigmentation—Although rare, multiple diffuse melanotic pigmentations can occur in HIV-infected subjects.

Hemochromatosis—This disease can be inherited or acquired and represents excessive deposition of iron pigments in the skin and mucosa. Melanosis is also an accompaniment because of adrenal involvement in the disease with secondary addisonian features.

Acanthosis nigricans—This is a cutaneous lesion that may occur on the face or lips and is associated with adenocarcinoma of the intestinal tract. The lesions are papillary and pigmented black and brown as a result of basilar melanosis.

PURPURA (PETECHIAE, ECCHYMOSES)

Coagulation factor deficiencies—Chronic liver failure of any cause results in deficient synthesis of clotting factors. In sprue or steatorrhea and in biliary cirrhosis, malabsorption of fat, including fat-soluble vitamin K, results in deficient clotting factor synthesis. The inherited factor deficiencies also lead to ecchymosis, which can be seen in the oral cavity or on the facial skin.

Thrombocytopenia—A decrease in platelets occurs in autoimmune disease because of the formation of antiplatelet antibodies. In addition, any disease process that destroys or replaces hematopoietic marrow can cause anemia, leukopenia, and thrombocytopenia. The more common ones include leukemia, myeloma, primary lymphoma of bone, metastatic cancer in bone, and chemotherapeutic drugs. Clinically, petechial hemorrhages are seen; when oral mucosa is involved, cutaneous lesions are usually evident as well.

Thrombocytopathia—Defective platelet function with inability to adhere to vessel walls or aggregate with one another occurs in heritable defects of adhesion. Von Willebrand's disease is the most common of these disorders. Clinically, petechial hemorrhages are seen; when oral mucosa is involved, cutaneous lesions are usually evident as well.

Infectious mononucleosis—Palatal petechiae can occur and are probably caused by suction of the soft palate against the base of the tongue as the patient attempts to palliate his or her itchy or sore throat.

MYCOTIC INFECTIONS

Candidiasis—Patients with diabetes mellitus, HIV infection, or various other diseases involving immunocompromise (e.g., leukemia, lymphoma, T-cell deficiencies, chronic granulomatous disease of childhood, DiGeorge's syndrome) are prone to develop oral candidiasis. The oral lesions are white, red, or mixed.

Invasive fungi—Histoplasmosis and blastomycosis can become disseminated from pulmonary foci. Cryptococcosis as well as the other rare fungal infections can occur in immunocompromised patients. The oral lesions appear as granular ulcerations.

Mucormycosis—Phycomycetosis occurs most often in brittle insulin-dependent diabetics and in immunocompromised patients. The maxillary sinus is the most common site, and ulceration through the maxillary alveolus and palate may occur.

ULCERATIVE AND VESICULAR LESIONS

Viral infection—Oral vesiculoulcerative lesions may occur in systemic viral infection, including primary varicella-zoster, measles, and hand, foot, and mouth coxsackievirus infection.

Agranulocytosis, neutropenia—Bone marrow suppression can be idiopathic, as in aplastic anemia, or secondary to lesions that infiltrate the hematopoietic marrow (myelophthisic anemia). Leukemia, lymphoma, myeloma, and carcinoma metastatic to bone are the main diseases. A painful ulcerative stomatitis may occur in conjunction with the decrease in granulocytes.

Cyclic neutropenia—An episodic defect in neutrophil maturation occurs in cyclic neutropenia, a heritable disease of childhood. The neutropenia persists only for a few days each month and may be followed by short-duration oral ulcerations.

Gluten enteropathy—An allergic reaction to gliadin in wheat is the cause of a malabsorption syndrome characterized by steatorrhea and dermatitis herpetiformis in the skin. Oral aphthous-like ulcerations also occur in this disease.

Chronic inflammatory bowel disease—Patients with ulcerative colitis may manifest recurrent, aphthous-like oral ulcerations.

HIV infection—Persistent, large, single or multiple ulcers similar to major aphthae are seen in some HIV-infected patients.

Behçet's syndrome—Rheumatoid arthritis, genital ulceration, and oral aphthous-like ulcerations are the characteristic features of this immunologic disease. The oral ulcers are often large and persistent, resembling those seen in major aphthae.

Uremia—In severe end-stage renal disease, oral ulcerations may be seen. Their origin has been associated with high ammonia levels in saliva.

Granulomatous infections—Large ulcers, focal or multiple, may be seen in tuberculosis and invasive fungal infections. The oral lesions represent a focus from widespread disseminated infection. In addition, chancre of primary syphilis may occur in oral mucosa or on the lip.

BULLOUS–DESQUAMATIVE DISEASES

Pemphigus vulgaris—Thirty percent of pemphigus cases begin in oral mucosa. The bullae can occur anywhere but are most often seen on the soft palate.

Erythema multiforme—Most cases of erythema multiforme affect both skin and mucosa. Skin lesions are either bullous or target configurations; the most severely affected oral sites are the lips.

Bullous pemphigoid—This skin disease may occasionally show bullae in the oral mucosa. Mucous membrane pemphigoid, with few exceptions, is restricted to mucous membranes and is a separate entity.

Pyostomatitis vegetans—In ulcerative colitis, a vegetative skin eruption may occur (pyodermatitis vegetante), and its oral counterpart appears as diffuse pebbly erosions and desquamations.

WHITE LESIONS

Lichen planus—Although often restricted to oral mucosa, lichen planus is also associated with keratotic skin lesions that tend to occur on the wrists. The oral lesions are reticular, plaque-like, or erosive, and the buccal mucosa and vestibule are favored sites.

Lupus erythematosus—Oral and labial white, red, or erosive plaques may be seen in both discoid and systemic lupus. They frequently present with perilesional fringe or striae. Oral lesions in the absence of skin plaques are rare.

Keratosis follicularis—In this heritable defect in the keratinization process, hyperkeratotic plaques occur on the skin. In the oral cavity, the lesions are white and pebbly, resembling a cobblestone street.

Secondary syphilis—Mucous patches of secondary syphilis may accompany the maculopapular rash. They occur on the lips and buccal mucosa as smooth flat circular white patches.

RED LESIONS

(See also sections on ulcerative and vesicular lesions, bullous–desquamative diseases, mycotic infections, and purpura.)

Pernicious anemia and folate deficiency—In these anemias, a bald, red, smooth tongue is seen. The normal tongue papillae have undergone atrophy.

SOFT TISSUE SWELLINGS

Regional enteritis (Crohn's disease)—Granulomatous inflammation of the bowel is sometimes heralded by the presence of oral mucosal granulomas. They appear as submucosal nodules and may be multinodular. Most occur in the buccal mucosa and vestibule.

Acanthosis nigricans—A cutaneous lesion that can occur on the face or lips; acanthosis nigricans is associated with adenocarcinoma of the intestinal tract. The lesions are papillary and pigmented black and brown because of basilar melanosis.

Metastatic carcinoma—Breast, lung, colon, and thyroid cancers are the most common to metastasize. They usually appear in the mandible but can occur as soft tissue swellings anywhere in the mouth.

Leukemia and lymphoma—Leukemic infiltrates, particularly in myelogenous leukemia, occur in the gingiva, producing diffuse enlargement of the papillae. Lymphomas may arise in the oral cavity or represent a focus of disseminated disease. A soft diffuse swelling of the hard and soft palates is the most common presentation for lymphoma.

Wegener's granulomatosis—Pulmonary, oropharyngeal, and nasal involvement with vasculitis is observed in Wegener's granulomatosis. Diffuse red and granular gingival enlargement is typical, and the nasal mucosa may also show granulomas.

Invasive fungi—Histoplasmosis and blastomycosis may become disseminated from pulmonary foci. Cryptococcosis as well as other fungal infections can occur in immunocompromised patients. The oral lesions appear as granular ulcerations.

Amyloidosis—The pathologic glycoprotein amyloid is deposited in primary amyloidosis and secondarily in myeloma, tuberculosis, and some dialysis patients. Oral lesions are nodules and can occur anywhere; the tongue and gingiva are most often involved.

Cowden syndrome—Multiple hamartomas of the skin, breast, mucosa, and thyroid occur in this hereditary condition. Breast carcinoma is a risk. The oral lesions are usually seen on the gingiva and appear as diffuse papular or papillary enlargements.

Multiple endocrine neoplasia (MEN) syndrome—Type III MEN involves the oral and conjunctival mucosae. Pheochromocytoma and medullary carcinoma of the thyroid are the two endocrine tumors that occur. The oral lesions are characterized by multiple small nodules of the anterior tongue and lips. These nodules are neuromatous tissue.

Neurofibromatosis (von Recklinghausen's disease of the skin)—This heritable disease is characterized by multiple skin nodules or pendulous tumors and brown macular pigmentations that may involve the head and neck skin. Intraoral café-au-lait pigmentation is rare.

HEAD AND NECK SWELLINGS

Infections—Systemic infections are often associated with cervical adenopathy and include HIV infection, mononucleosis, cat-scratch fever, and scrofula.

Malignancy—Disseminated cancers with cervical swelling are lymphomas of both Hodgkin's and non-Hodgkin's types.

Sjögren's syndrome—Bilateral parotid enlargement with xerostomia, xerophthalmia, and rheumatoid arthritis are classic components. Secondary Sjögren's syndrome can occur in conjunction with other collagen/immune diseases.

Sarcoidosis—Involvement of the lips occurs in the Melkersson-Rosenthal syndrome, whereas bilateral parotid involvement is seen in Heerfordt's syndrome. Although the granulomatous swellings are identical to those in systemic sarcoidosis, the face is often the only area affected in these two syndromes.

Cushing's syndrome—Diffuse facial edema (moon facies) occurs in adrenocortical hyperplasia and in patients on long-term steroid therapy.

Angioedema—Familial angioedema is characterized by diffuse lip and facial swelling with multiple foci of urticaria. It is caused by an enzyme deficiency involving one of the complement factors (C1 esterase inhibitor).

INTRAOSSEOUS JAW LESIONS

Hyperparathyroidism—A ground-glass appearance of the alveolar bone may be seen, and multilocular radiolucencies representing giant cell lesions (brown tumors) can arise in the jaws in both primary and secondary (renal) hyperparathyroidism.

Osteitis deformans—Paget's disease of bone is polyostotic and usually affects the jaws, most often the maxilla. Hypercementosis may be seen, and the alveolar bone is expanded, with ground-glass opacification early in the disease and cotton-wool confluent opacities later.

Fibrous dysplasia—Most instances of fibrous dysplasia in the maxillofacial complex are monostotic. About 5% are polyostotic, warranting a skeletal survey. Albright's syndrome—characterized by polyostotic fibrous dysplasia, precocious puberty, thyroid enlargement, and café-au-lait pigmentation of the skin—is extremely rare.

Multiple myeloma—Disseminated plasma cell myeloma causes lytic bone lesions and can be seen in the jaws and skull bones as coin-shaped punched-out radiolucencies. Pain is common.

Metastatic carcinoma—Breast, lung, colon, and thyroid cancers are the most common to metastasize. Most often they appear in the mandible, where they invade the inferior alveolar nerve, causing lip paresthesia and a detectable radiolucency or mixed radiolucent and radiopaque lesion.

Gardner's syndrome—Premalignant intestinal polyps are the main component of this syndrome. Other abnormalities include desmoid tumors of the skin; cutaneous cysts; osteomas of the skull, jaws, and sinuses; and supernumerary teeth.

Osteopetrosis—Marble bone disease is a defect in osteoclastic activity such that osteogenesis, during development, goes unchecked and unremodeled. In dental radiographs, the alveolar bone is so dense that the roots are obscured. This opacification is generalized throughout the skeleton, with an attending myelophthisic anemia. Osteomyelitis of the jaws secondary to odontogenic infection is a complication in this extremely rare disease.

Caffey's disease—Infantile cortical hyperostosis of Caffey is associated with bone tenderness, intestinal distress, and irritability among infants under 1 year of age. Mandibular enlargement with radiographic evidence of cortical redundancy is encountered. The disorder probably represents an osseous growth spurt during the course of development.

PERIODONTAL BONE DESTRUCTION

Diabetes mellitus—Particularly in the insulin-dependent form, periodontitis is severe and periodontal abscesses are common, probably as a result of the microvascular disease in the periodontal ligament.

HIV infection—A specific form of periodontal disease affects some patients who are infected with HIV. The lesions occur without pocket formation since both hard and soft periodontal tissues undergo rapid necrosis. The lesions tend to be multifocal with intervening normal gingiva.

Langerhans' cell histiocytosis—Infiltration of various tissues by histiocytes (also termed *histiocytosis X*) occurs in this disease. Retroorbital involvement causes exophthalmos; posterior pituitary involvement results in diabetes insipidus. Jaw involvement is characterized by radiolucencies that surround teeth and are often multifocal. A "tooth floating in space" appearance is often encountered radiographically.

Scleroderma—A minority of patients with systemic sclerosis show widened periodontal ligament spaces on radiographs. This change is a component of the widespread collagenization of the soft tissues and does not predispose to periodontal disease. Alternatively, scleroderma patients are prone to develop microstomia and mucogingival defects because of scarring of the submucosa.

DENTAL ALTERATIONS IN SYSTEMIC DISEASE

Amelogenesis imperfecta—This may occur in conjunction with other syndromes and conditions, including the mucopolysaccharidoses, oculodento-osseous dysplasia, amelo-onycho-hypohidrotic syndrome, and trichodento-osseous syndrome.

Dentinogenesis imperfecta—This defect in dentin formation is often associated with osteogenesis imperfecta. Blue sclerae are seen.

Enamel erosion—If enamel erosion is localized to the lingual and palatal surfaces of the teeth, anorexia or bulimia should be suspected.

Enamel pitting—Multiple small enamel pits may occur in tuberous sclerosis and certain forms of epidermolysis bullosa.

Pigmentation of teeth—A variety of systemic diseases can cause dental discoloration. Congenital jaundice due to biliary atresia or erythroblastosis fetalis deposits bilirubin pigments in teeth. Other iron-transporting molecules (porphyrins) may accumulate in developing teeth among patients with porphyria. Fluoride ingestion also causes brown and chalky white discoloration but usually has no other adverse systemic manifestations.

Ectodermal dysplasia—In this inherited X-linked recessive disease, skin adnexal structures, including hair follicles and sweat glands, fail to develop. Teeth are also missing, but the cuspids usually form and show conical crowns.

Chondroectodermal dysplasia (Ellis–van Creveld syndrome)—Both epidermal and mesenchymal tissues are defective. Missing and malformed teeth are encountered.

Incontinentia pigmenti—This is an X-linked genetic disease that is lethal in affected males. Affected girls manifest multisystem anomalies with oligodontia, conical crowns, and delayed eruption.

Epidermolysis bullosa—Thin enamel with pitting is encountered in some forms of inherited epidermolysis bullosa.

Hypophosphatasia—This is caused by an inborn error of metabolism with defective osteogenesis and cementogenesis due to a lack of the enzyme alkaline phosphatase, which is responsible for phosphorylation of bone matrix. Teeth lack cementum and are prematurely exfoliated.

Vitamin D–refractory rickets—In this inherited disease, a defective enzyme prevents the conversion of vitamin D to its active form. Teeth show enlarged coronal pulp chambers with coronal defects through the dentin, which appear as large pulp horns. Enamel pitting and defects are also encountered.

Taurodontism—Anomalous teeth with large pulp chambers are encountered in the trichodento-osseous syndrome.

Pseudohypoparathyroidism—Two forms of this inherited disease exist, both involving males. There is a failure to eliminate phosphate in the kidneys. Many abnormalities, including round facies, short neck, cerebral calcifications, short digits, and enamel pitting of the premolars and molars, are encountered.

Cleidocranial dysplasia—Clavicles fail to develop, and supernumerary impacted teeth are present.

Gardner's syndrome—Premalignant intestinal polyps are the main component of this syndrome. Other abnormalities include desmoid tumors of the skin; cutaneous cysts; osteomas of the skull, jaws, and sinuses; and supernumerary teeth.

SENSORY DEFICITS

Burning tongue and mucosa—When no lesions are observed, anemias and diabetes should be considered and investigated. In most cases, the symptom is associated with chronic depressive illness.

Paresthesia—Paresthesia occurs in metastatic carcinoma to the mandible, osteitis deformans, multiple sclerosis, and diabetes.

Dysgeusia—Distortion of the sense of taste may develop from stroke and with renal disease, sinus disease, influenza, and zinc deficiency.

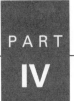

PART

IV

Pain and Neuromuscular Disorders

ACUTE FACIAL PAIN*

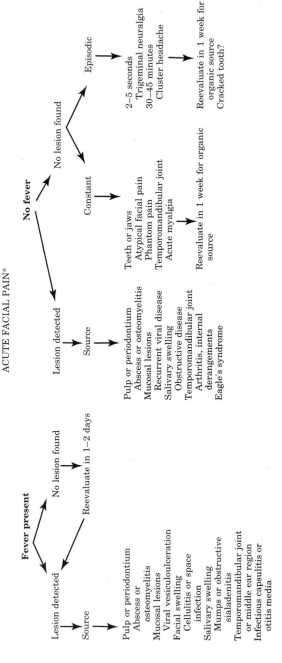

Fever present

No lesion found → Reevaluate in 1–2 days

Lesion detected → Source →
- Pulp or periodontium
- Abscess or osteomyelitis
- Mucosal lesions
- Viral vesiculoulceration
- Facial swelling
- Cellulitis or space infection
- Salivary swelling
- Mumps or obstructive sialadenitis
- Temporomandibular joint or middle ear region
- Infectious capsulitis or otitis media

No fever

Lesion detected → Source →
- Pulp or periodontium
- Abscess or osteomyelitis
- Mucosal lesions
- Recurrent viral disease
- Salivary swelling
- Obstructive disease
- Temporomandibular joint
- Arthritis, internal derangements
- Eagle's syndrome

No lesion found →

Constant →
- Teeth or jaws
- Atypical facial pain
- Phantom pain
- Temporomandibular joint
- Acute myalgia

→ Reevaluate in 1 week for organic source

Episodic →
- 2–5 seconds Trigeminal neuralgia
- 30–45 minutes Cluster headache

→ Reevaluate in 1 week for organic source
Cracked tooth?

*These are the most likely entities to be considered. Other rare and esoteric diseases can also cause pain.

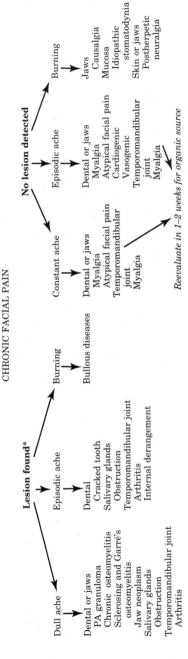

CHRONIC FACIAL PAIN

Lesion found*

Dull ache

Dental or jaws
PA granuloma
Chronic osteomyelitis
Sclerosing and Garré's osteomyelitis
Jaw neoplasm
Salivary glands
Obstruction
Temporomandibular joint
Arthritis

Episodic ache

Dental
Cracked tooth
Salivary glands
Obstruction
Temporomandibular joint
Arthritis
Internal derangement

Burning

Bullous diseases

No lesion detected

Constant ache

Dental or jaws
Myalgia
Atypical facial pain
Temporomandibular joint
Myalgia

Episodic ache

Dental or jaws
Myalgia
Atypical facial pain
Cardiogenic
Vasogenic
Temporomandibular joint
Myalgia

Burning

Jaws
Causalgia
Mucosa
Idiopathic stomatodynia
Skin or jaws
Postherpetic neuralgia

Reevaluate in 1–2 weeks for organic source

Lesions include caries, radiographic changes, swellings, erosions, joint sounds, and so forth.

Pain

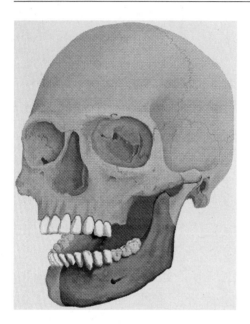

SUSTAINED ACUTE MANDIBULAR PAIN

Acute pulpitis
Apical abscess
Acute or subacute osteomyelitis

Significant Findings

1. Sensitivity to heat, cold, and palpation
2. Elevated temperature
3. Fistula, parulis, or extraoral drainage tracts may be seen in apical abscess and osteomyelitis.

Diagnostic Procedures

1. Pulp testing with hot and cold stimuli, percussion, and vitalometry uncovers odontogenic infections.
2. Percussion sensitivity indicates apical infection.
3. Periapical radiographic examination can detect odontogenic infection. Panoramic films disclose a diffuse radiolucency, usually moth-eaten in appearance, in osteomyelitis.
4. Culture and sensitivity should be tested when drainage is seen.

Management

1. Localized acute odontogenic infection requires root canal therapy or extraction. Any parulis can be incised and drained.
2. Osteomyelitis requires long-term antibiotic therapy. Incision and drainage with local osseous debridement may be necessary in severe cases. Failure to resolve warrants reculture, including anaerobe assessment and sensitivity testing.

EPISODIC ACUTE MANDIBULAR PAIN

Acute pulpitis
Apical abscess
Cracked tooth
Coronary artery disease
Trigeminal neuralgia
Eagle's syndrome

Significant Findings

1. When a specific tooth can be identified, an odontogenic infection or a cracked tooth should be suspected.
2. Precipitating factors should be explored. Cold sensitivity points to an odontogenic source; pain on exertion should arouse suspicion of coronary artery disease, particularly if a substernal component exists. A trigger point is seen in trigeminal neuralgia; twisting the head and neck impinges on a cracked calcified stylohyoid ligament in Eagle's syndrome; and lateral pressure on cusp inclines causes pain in a cracked tooth.
3. Severe acute lancinating or electrical paroxysms lasting only seconds characterize trigeminal neuralgia.

Diagnostic Procedures

1. Pulp testing with hot and cold stimuli, percussion, and vitalometry can uncover odontogenic infections.
2. Percussion sensitivity indicates apical infection.
3. Occlusion on an instrument with lateral pressure is used to test for cracked teeth.
4. Blood pressure recording of hypertension may suggest coronary artery disease, although such patients can be normotensive. In suspected coronary disease, medical referral for definitive diagnosis is required.
5. Periapical radiographic examination can detect odontogenic infection; panoramic films are needed to find calcified stylohyoid ligaments in patients with pain exacerbation on turning the head to the affected side.

Management

1. Odontogenic infections are treated with antibiotics, endodontics, or extraction.
2. Cracked teeth require bands, crowns, endodontics, or extraction.
3. Trigeminal neuralgia resolves with carbamazepine therapy, neurosurgery, or thermal nucleolysis.
4. Appropriate dietary and medical therapy must be undertaken for coronary disease.
5. Eagle's syndrome requires surgical removal of the fractured calcified ligament.

CHRONIC MANDIBULAR PAIN

Chronic apical periodontitis
Chronic osteomyelitis (sclerosing and Garré's)
Masseteric or pterygoid myalgia
Atypical facial pain

Significant Findings

1. History of pain symptoms and localization by patient often leads to the correct diagnosis, particularly if the patient can localize the pain to a specific tooth. Pain related to myalgia and osteomyelitis may be more diffuse and not localized.
2. Physical examination reveals percussion pain, jaw expansion, or palpation tenderness in odontogenic infection; trigger point tenderness of the masticatory muscles is seen in myalgic pain.
3. History of extraction or root canal therapy is common in patients with atypical facial pain, although no infectious source can be identified.

Diagnostic Procedures

1. Pulp vitality testing is needed for necrosis and odontogenic infection.
2. Periapical and panoramic films can detect periapical lesions indicative of granuloma, cyst, or osteomyelitis. Occlusal films are required for suspected periostitis.
3. Diagnostic drug trials (anxiolytics, muscle relaxants) can be tried for suspected myalgia.
4. When all physical sources are ruled out, atypical facial pain is the diagnosis by default.
5. Diagnostic selective block and infiltration anesthesia can be used to determine the precise location of the pain.

Management

1. Root canal therapy and antibiotics are needed for odontogenic infection.

2. Myalgia is treated by occlusal splint therapy, muscle relaxation exercises, physical therapy, and stress management strategies.
3. Atypical facial pain is recalcitrant to most therapies. Regional steroid injections, exploration for necrotizing cavitational lesions, and antidepressants have some utility.

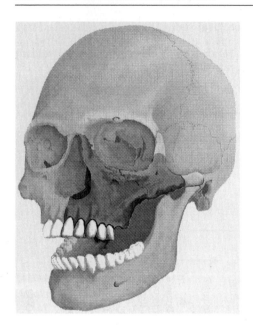

SUSTAINED ACUTE MAXILLARY PAIN

Acute pulpitis
Apical abscess
Periodontal abscess
Bacterial sinusitis

Significant Findings

1. Pain is usually severe and throbbing, keeping the patient awake at night.
2. Elevated temperature indicates acute infection.
3. Clinical endodontic testing for pulp vitality and sensitivity to heat, cold, and percussion is necessary. Heat or cold sensitivity indicates pulpitis; percussion sensitivity in a nonvital tooth reveals apical periodontitis.
4. Periodontal probing of pocket with expression of pus in a vital tooth reveals periodontal abscess. If the tooth is nonvital, combination endodontic and periodontal infection is the cause.
5. Sinusitis is revealed by percussion sensitivity of the maxillary posterior teeth, malar region percussion tenderness, nasal discharge, gravitational accentuation of pain (when the head is placed below the knees with the patient in a sitting position), and negative dental findings.

Diagnostic Procedures

1. Endodontic and periodontal diagnostic assessment should be undertaken as stated above.
2. Radiographic examination is revealing as follows:
   a. Deep dental caries indicate pulpitis.
   b. Periapical radiolucency or widened apical periodontal ligament indicates apical abscess.
   c. Alveolar bone loss, particularly vertical, is indicative of periodontal abscess.
   d. Nasal stuffiness or discharge with sinus opacification or air/fluid level points to sinusitis.

Management

1. Pulpitis or apical abscess requires endodontic therapy for restorable teeth or extraction for nonrestorable teeth. Antibiotic therapy is necessary when the patient's temperature is elevated because of lymphadenopathy. Analgesics may be needed.
2. Periodontal abscess requires incision, drainage, root planning, and curettage. Antibiotic therapy is needed when the patient's temperature is elevated because of lymphadenopathy. Analgesics may be needed.
3. Sinusitis necessitates antibiotic therapy, analgesics if needed, and referral to an ear, nose, and throat physician. Sinus lavage is necessary in some instances.

EPISODIC ACUTE MAXILLARY PAIN

Acute pulpitis
Cracked tooth
Cluster headache
Trigeminal neuralgia

Significant Findings

1. Pain comes and goes and is usually severe.
2. Acute pulpitis is indicated by a history of acute pain episodes when eating hot, cold, or sweet foods, or pain that lingers after application of ice to suspected tooth.
3. Sharp pain during mastication is indicative of a cracked tooth.
4. Acute episodes in the evening, often seasonal; ipsilateral conjunctival reddening with nasal discharge; and duration of 30 to 40 minutes indicate vascular cluster headache.
5. Severe electrical stabbing pain lasting only seconds with a trigger zone on the skin or in the mouth are typical features of trigeminal neuralgia.

Diagnostic Procedures

1. Radiographs to assess dental caries.
2. Endodontic testing is used to detect sensitivity to heat and cold that lingers, indicative of pulpitis.
3. Occlusion against a tongue blade or lateral pressure against cusps induces pain when the tooth is cracked. Fiberoptic assessment for cracks can also be diagnostic. Sometimes existing restorations must be removed to locate tooth fractures in the crown.
4. When all clinical and radiographic findings are negative for dental pathology, neuralgic syndromes should be suspected. Cluster headache and trigeminal neuralgia manifest unique clinical findings as listed above.
5. Administration of oxygen at the onset of a cluster headache often eliminates the pain, a finding of diagnostic significance.

Management

1. For pulpitis, endodontic therapy is used for restorable teeth, but extraction is necessary for nonrestorable teeth. Antibiotic therapy is required when the patient's temperature is elevated. Analgesics may be needed.
2. For cracked teeth, root fracture requires extraction. Some coronal fractures can be saved with full crown coverage or circumcoronal banding.
3. Classic cluster headaches occur daily or every other day for about 2 months, then clear. During pain episodes, calcium channel blockers usually prevent the vasoactive events that are thought to cause pain.
4. Endodontic therapy and extraction should be avoided in trigeminal neuralgia. Medical treatment with carbamazepine is effective, but blood counts must be monitored. Thermal nucleolysis of the ganglion is effective for patients whose condition cannot be managed medically.

CHRONIC MAXILLARY PAIN

Chronic apical periodontitis
Chronic (allergic) sinusitis
Masseteric myalgia
Atypical facial pain

Significant Findings

1. Palpation tenderness may indicate the origin of chronic pain. Tenderness may be felt in the alveolus in odontogenic infection; the malar region in sinusitis, or the muscles of mastication in myalgia. There is an absence of palpation tenderness in atypical facial pain.

2. Gravity (placing the head below the knees) worsens pain of sinus origin.
3. Disorders of affect (e.g., depression, anxiety, obsessive or compulsive personality disorder) may underlie atypical facial pain when no identifiable organic source can be found.
4. History of jaw clenching from anxiety suggests myalgia.
5. Seasonal onset (spring or fall) suggests sinusitis.

Diagnostic Procedures

1. Panoramic and periapical radiographic films can detect dental, periapical, or periodontal infection. Waters sinus radiographs, sinus tomograms, and computed tomography scans are utilized for sinusitis. No radiographic evidence of disease is seen in atypical facial pain.
2. Muscle palpation tenderness in myalgic pain referred to the maxilla is usually localized to the muscle origin over the malar eminence.
3. Muscle trigger point injection relieves pain in myalgia.
4. Tooth percussion tenderness is usually localized in odontogenic infection. In sinusitis, the entire posterior sextant is usually tender to percussion. The malar region is often tender to percussion in sinusitis.
5. Transillumination of the sinuses often discloses clouding in sinusitis.
6. When atypical facial pain or atypical odontalgia is the foremost consideration, psychologic, psychometric, and psychiatric evaluation should be considered.
7. In edentulous regions with no radiologic evidence of disease and no other significant clinical findings, diagnostic anesthesia should be undertaken to evaluate for symptom relief.

Management

1. Odontogenic and periodontal sources should be treated by endodontic therapy, extraction, or curettage as appropriate.
2. Patients with chronic sinusitis should be referred to an ear, nose, and throat specialist. Treatment consists of antihistamines, antibiotics, and sinus lavage.
3. Atypical facial pain and odontalgia are difficult to manage. Most patients insist their problems are organic despite negative physical findings. Referral to a counselor, psychologist, or psychiatrist is recommended.
4. Myalgia can be managed by many strategies, including stress management, biofeedback, trigger-point injections of bupivacaine (Marcaine), acrylic splints, and psychologic counseling.

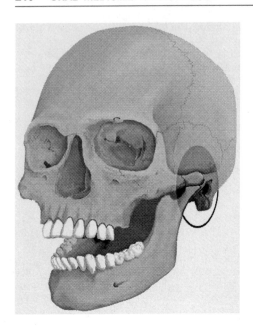

ACUTE TEMPOROMANDIBULAR JOINT REGION ARTHRALGIA

Capsulitis or synovitis
Trauma
Infectious arthritis
Masticatory myalgia
Odontogenic infection
Otitis media

Significant Findings

1. Pain over the joint is encountered in joint inflammation but not in otitis. In myalgia, the pain is more diffuse and generalized over the masseteric and temporalis regions.
2. A history of injury is obviously of diagnostic importance.
3. In acute infectious processes of the joint or middle ear, cervical lymphadenopathy may be observed and the patient is usually febrile.
4. All of these disorders may manifest deviant or limited opening, although such signs are not often encountered in otitis.
5. Unilateral hearing impairment is a feature of otitis.
6. Trigger point tenderness is indicative of myalgia.
7. Anxiety with severe sustained tooth clenching also suggests myalgia.

Diagnostic Procedures

1. Joint palpation tenderness indicates a synovial, capsular, or arthritic disease process.
2. Otoscopic examination can disclose a bulging, perforated, purulent, red or telangiectatic tympanic membrane in otitis media.
3. Pulp testing and vitalometry of posterior teeth should be considered. Referred pain in the temporomandibular joint may evolve from an infected second or third molar.
4. Aspiration of the capsule in acute capsulitis or synovitis yields a purulent exudate that should be subjected to culture and sensitivity testing.

Management

1. Acute capsulitis or synovitis requires incision and drainage. Antibiotic therapy with analgesics (a narcotic for moderate pain level).
2. A patient with otitis media should be referred to an ear, nose, and throat specialist.
3. An odontogenic source is treated by endodontics, extraction, or periodontal curettage, depending on the precise nature of the infection. Antibiotics and analgesics are also indicated.
4. Acute myalgia can be treated by trigger-point bupivacaine (Marcaine) injections, physical therapy, and prescription of muscle relaxants and analgesics.

CHRONIC TEMPOROMANDIBULAR JOINT REGION ARTHRALGIA

Internal derangement of the meniscus
Capsular adhesions
Arthritides
Myalgia
Neoplasia

Significant Findings

1. Pain localized precisely in the condylar region is indicative of an organic lesion in the joint itself; more diffuse pain over the masseter and temporalis is more typical for myalgia.
2. If there is swelling over the condyle, neoplasia should be suspected if it is firm or indulated. Fluctuant swelling indicates infectious arthritis or synovitis.
3. A click in the joint is consistent with internal derangement with displaced meniscus; crepitus indicates bone erosions secondary to arthritis.
4. Limited opening indicates bilateral disease; deviant opening is consistent with unilateral disease (jaw deviates toward the affected side).

5. A history of sustained chronic tooth clenching indicates probable myalgia.

Diagnostic Procedures

1. Stethoscope assessment of joint sounds is undertaken for clicking or crepitus.
2. Pain on joint palpation is indicative of inflammatory joint disease. Acute pain indicates possible bacterial infection.
3. Arthroscopy can disclose erosions, meniscus displacement, and adhesions in arthritis, as well as internal derangements of the enveloping tissues.
4. Tomograms of the temporomandibular joint can disclose osseous changes in the arthritides. Magnetic resonance imaging can show meniscus displacement. Computed tomography or magnetic resonance imaging can define neoplastic conditions of the joint and capsule.
5. Administration of intravenous diazepam (valium) with manual manipulation of the mandible can identify limited opening due to myalgia. Under intravenous sedation, the jaw can generally be manually manipulated without impedance.

Management

1. Internal derangements can usually be managed with nonsteroidal anti-inflammatory drugs (NSAIDs), acrylic splints, and physical therapy. Severe pain symptoms and response failure to noninvasive treatments constitute a consideration for surgical correction (meniscectomy, meniscus plication).
2. Chronic myalgia can be treated by NSAIDs, muscle relaxants, physical therapy, and psychologic counseling with stress management and biofeedback.
3. Arthritides are treated with NSAIDs and physical therapy. When severe pain symptoms cannot be resolved by these methods, surgery may be considered.
4. Neoplasms and reactive proliferations of the temporomandibular joint and associated tissues are rare and include such benign lesions as nodular synovitis, osteochondroma, and giant cell tumors of the tendon sheath, which are treated by local excision. Malignant tumors include synovial sarcoma and contiguous salivary adenocarcinomas and require radical excision of the tumor, the condyle, and the temporal bone.

Limited and Deviant Jaw Opening

TRISMUS

Internal derangement of the meniscus
Capsular adhesions

Arthritides
Myalgia
Neoplasia
Odontogenic infection
Coronoid hyperplasia

Significant Findings

1. Pain localized precisely in the condylar region is indicative of an organic lesion in the joint itself; more-diffuse pain over the masseter and temporalis is typical for myalgia. Vague pain over the joint and ramus suggests odontogenic origin.
2. If there is swelling over the condyle, neoplasia should be suspected if the swelling is firm or indulated. Fluctuant swelling indicates infectious arthritis or synovitis. Swelling in the retromolar area with operculitis indicates trismus from infection of a partially impacted tooth follicle.
3. A click in the joint is consistent with internal derangement with displaced meniscus; crepitus indicates bone erosions secondary to arthritis.
4. Limited opening indicates bilateral disease; deviant opening is consistent with unilateral disease (jaw deviates toward the affected side).
5. Anxiety with tooth clenching contributes to myalgia.

Diagnostic Procedures

1. Stethoscope assessment of joint sounds for clicking or crepitus.
2. Pain on joint palpation is indicative of inflammatory joint disease. Acute pain indicates possible bacterial infection.
3. Arthroscopy can disclose erosions, meniscus displacement, and adhesions in arthritis, as well as internal derangements of the enveloping tissues.
4. Panoramic and periapical films can disclose odontogenic infections as periapical or pericoronal radiolucencies (the latter in the case of an infected follicle). Temporomandibular joint tomograms can disclose osseous changes in the arthritides and, along with plain films, can show coronoid enlargement in coronoid hyperplasia. Magnetic resonance imaging can demonstrate meniscus displacements. Computed tomography or magnetic resonance imaging can define neoplastic conditions of the joint and capsule.
5. Pulp and vitalometry testing is necessary to check for a pulpal source of infection; periodontal probing for pericoronal or periodontal abscess.
6. Administration of intravenous valium with manual manipulation of the mandible can usually identify limited opening due to myalgia. Under intravenous sedation, the jaw can generally be manually manipulated without impedance.

Management

1. Internal derangements can usually be managed with NSAIDs, acrylic splints, and physical therapy. Severe pain symptoms and failure to resolve after noninvasive treatments constitute a consideration for surgical correction (meniscectomy, meniscus plication).

2. Chronic myalgia can be treated by NSAIDs, muscle relaxants, physical therapy, and psychologic counseling with stress management and biofeedback.

3. Extraction of wisdom teeth may be necessary in pericoronitis or operculitis; endodontic therapy or extraction is required for other odontogenic infections. Periodontal curettage should be undertaken for periodontal abscesses, and analgesics and antibiotics should be prescribed.

4. Coronoidectomy is the treatment of choice for limited opening due to hyperplasia. Most instances are bilateral.

5. Neoplasms and reactive proliferations of the temporomandibular joint and associated tissues are rare and include such benign lesions as nodular synovitis, osteochondroma, and giant cell tumor of tendon sheath, which are treated by local excision. Malignant tumors include synovial sarcoma and contiguous salivary adenocarcinomas, which require radical excision of the tumor, the condyle, and the temporal bone.

DEVIATION

Internal derangement of the meniscus
Capsular adhesions
Arthritides
Myalgia
Neoplasia
Condylar hyperplasia

Significant Findings

1. Pain localized precisely in the condylar region is indicative of an organic lesion in the joint itself; more diffuse pain over the masseter and temporalis is typical for myalgia.

2. Neoplasia should be suspected if there is firm or indulated swelling over the condyle. Fluctuant swelling indicates infectious arthritis or synovitis.

3. A click in the joint is consistent with internal derangement with displaced meniscus; crepitus indicates bone erosions secondary to arthritis.

4. Deviant opening is consistent with unilateral disease (jaw deviates toward the affected side). When the jaw deviates then corrects to midline on full opening, a displaced disc should be suspected (reducing internal derangement). Deviation without correction indicates unilateral closed lock and can be seen in any of these conditions.

5. A posterior open bite on the same side as the direction of deviation and affected joint is indicative of unilateral condylar hyperplasia.

Diagnostic Procedures

1. Stethoscope assessment of joint sounds for clicking or crepitus.
2. Pain on joint palpation is indicative of inflammatory joint disease. Acute pain indicates possible bacterial infection.
3. Arthroscopy can disclose erosions, meniscus displacement, and adhesions in arthritis, as well as internal derangements of the enveloping tissues.
4. Tomograms of the temporomandibular joint can disclose osseous changes in the arthritides and evidence of condylar enlargement in condylar hyperplasias. Magnetic resonance imaging can show meniscus displacements. Plain films can also show condylar enlargement. Computed tomography or magnetic resonance imaging can define neoplastic conditions of the joint and capsule.
5. Administration of intravenous valium with manual manipulation of the mandible usually identifies limited opening due to myalgia. Under intravenous sedation, the jaw can generally be manually manipulated without impedance.

Management

1. Internal derangements can usually be managed with NSAIDs, acrylic splints, and physical therapy. Severe pain symptoms without response to noninvasive treatments constitute a consideration for surgical correction (meniscectomy, meniscus plication).
2. Chronic myalgia can be treated by NSAIDs, muscle relaxants, physical therapy, and psychologic counseling with stress management and biofeedback.
3. Arthritides are treated with NSAIDs and physical therapy. When severe pain symptoms cannot be resolved by these methods, surgery should be considered.
4. Partial condylectomy or recontouring is the treatment of choice for deviant opening due to hyperplasia.
5. Neoplasms and reactive proliferations of the temporomandibular joint and associated tissues are rare and include such benign lesions as nodular synovitis, osteochondroma, and giant cell tumor of tendon sheath, which are treated by local excision. Malignant tumors include synovial sarcoma and contiguous salivary adenocarcinomas, which require radical excision of the tumor, the condyle, and the temporal bone.

Burning Mouth

STOMATODYNIA AND GLOSSODYNIA

Depressive illness
Sjögren's syndrome

Candidiasis
Radiation mucositis
Stomatitides

Significant Findings

1. Normal oral findings, history of personal or psychologic loss, early morning awakening, and anhedonia in an elderly adult, particularly a woman, often heralds psychologic depressive illness.
2. Inflamed-appearing erythematous mucosa with burning is usually attributable to organic disease: extreme dryness-radiation for head and neck cancer and Sjögren's syndrome; patchy appearance may suggest candida infection, rule out HIV and diabetes as predisposing factors.
3. Desquamations or ulcerations indicate viral and bullous stomatitides. See sections on vesicles, ulcers, and desquamations.

Diagnostic Procedures

1. Psychologic evaluation is needed for depression-associated stomatodynia. Antidepressant medications can be used as a therapeutic and diagnostic trial.
2. Cytologic smear is necessary for detection of candidal yeasts and mycelia.
3. Physical examination is used for detection of bilateral parotid involvement, xerophthalmia, and rheumatic joint disease. Specific functional tests are required to determine salivary output (flow rate) and lacrimation (Schirmer test). The Rose-Bengal dye assessment is employed for the diagnosis of keratoconjunctivitis sicca.
4. HIV serologic testing should be undertaken for unexplained candidal infection in high-risk patients. Serologic testing for rheumatoid factor and other autoantibodies detectable in Sjögren's syndrome and secondary Sjögren's syndrome that are associated with collagen/immune diseases should be undertaken, including SSA, anti-DNA, anti-Rho, and antinuclear antibodies.
5. Fasting blood sugar to determine the presence of diabetes in unexplained candidiasis.
6. For identification of erosions, bullae, desquamations, or ulcerations, see section on diagnosis of vesicular, desquamative, and ulcerative diseases.

Management

1. Burning mouth in the absence of any organic mucosal changes is usually manageable by prescription of antidepressant medications. Whether the symptom of stomatodynia is truly specific for depressive illness is unknown. However, most patients respond favorably within 4 or 5 weeks, but not usually before.

2. Xerostomia-associated burning is a complex management problem since patients with Sjögren's syndrome or those who have undergone radiation therapy are not able to regenerate salivary tissues. Salivary substitutes, transmucosal electrostimulation, and pilocarpine can all be of some benefit.
3. Candidiasis with burning erythematous mucosa can be treated with antifungals in conjunction with topical chlorhexidine mouth rinses. When underlying systemic diseases exist, such as diabetes and HIV, episodic recurrences are to be expected and can be treated periodically.

Dry Mouth

XEROSTOMIA

Drug-induced
Primary Sjögren's syndrome
Secondary Sjögren's syndrome
Radiation-induced
Idiopathic

Significant Findings

1. The primary cause of xerostomia is medications, so a history of drug use is of chief importance. The primary culprits are antihistamines, antidepressants, and antihypertensive agents, particularly diuretics.
2. In Sjögren's syndrome, xerophthalmia is a complaint, and physical examination often discloses parotid enlargement.
3. Secondary Sjögren's syndrome involves autoimmune parotitis that occurs with other collagen diseases such as rheumatoid arthritis, lupus, systemic sclerosis, and mixed collagen disease. Therefore, physical examination may disclose specific skin and joint lesions.
4. A history of head and neck cancer with radiation therapy explains the findings, since radiation exceeding 50 cGy induces acinar necrosis and fibrosis.

Diagnostic Procedures

1. Physical examination is used for detection of bilateral parotid involvement, xerophthalmia, and rheumatic joint disease. Specific functional tests are required to determine salivary output (flow rate) and lacrimation (Schirmer test). The Rose-Bengal dye assessment is employed to confirm keratoconjunctivitis sicca.
2. Serologic testing should be undertaken for rheumatoid factor and other autoantibodies detectable in Sjögren's syndrome and secondary Sjögren's syndrome that is associated with collagen/

immune diseases, including SSA, anti-DNA, anti-Rho, and antinuclear antibodies.
3. When Sjögren's syndrome is suspected, a lower lip biopsy specimen should be taken, with five or six minor salivary lobules harvested from the submucosa. Focus score assessment (number of lymphoid aggregates per salivary lobule) read by the pathologist as 2+ or greater corroborates the diagnosis of Sjögren's syndrome.

Management

1. Drug-related xerostomia can be minimized by lowering the dosage or changing the medication in consultation with the patient's physician. Nevertheless, the patient may have to adjust to the symptoms if no alternative medication can be found. Saliva substitutes may be of benefit in such instances.
2. Xerostomia-associated burning is a complex management problem since patients with Sjögren's syndrome or those who have undergone radiation therapy are not able to regenerate salivary tissues. Salivary substitutes, transmucosal electrostimulation, and pilocarpine therapy may all be of some benefit.
3. When all tests are negative, the diagnosis is idiopathic xerostomia. Psychosomatic origin must be considered and discussed with the patient, and he or she must be assured that no organic disease is present.

NEUROLOGIC DEFICITS

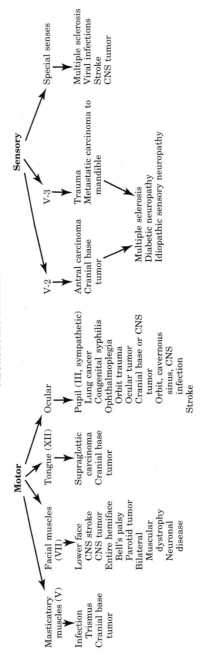

Motor

Masticatory muscles (V)
- Infection
- Trismus
- Cranial base tumor

Facial muscles (VII)
- Lower face
  - CNS stroke
  - CNS tumor
- Entire hemiface
  - Bell's palsy
  - Parotid tumor
- Bilateral
  - Muscular dystrophy
  - Neuronal disease

Tongue (XII)
- Supraglottic carcinoma
- Cranial base tumor

Ocular
- Pupil (III, sympathetic)
- Lung cancer
- Congenital syphilis
- Ophthalmoplegia
- Orbit trauma
- Ocular tumor
- Cranial base or CNS tumor
- Orbit, cavernous sinus, CNS infection
- Stroke

Sensory

V-2
- Antral carcinoma
- Cranial base tumor
  - Multiple sclerosis
  - Diabetic neuropathy
  - Idiopathic sensory neuropathy

V-3
- Trauma
- Metastatic carcinoma to mandible

Special senses
- Multiple sclerosis
- Viral infections
- Stroke
- CNS tumor

Paresthesia or Hypoesthesia (Sensory Deficit)

Nerve trauma due to mandibular third molar surgery
Viral paresthesia
Multiple sclerosis
Diabetic neuropathy
Carcinoma

Significant Findings

1. Localization is based on nerve V divisions: paresthesia of V2 suggests antral carcinoma; paresthesia of V3 suggests metastatic carcinoma to the mandible.
2. History of jaw fracture, third molar extraction, or oral surgery with paresthesia is indicative of nerve trauma.
3. Sudden onset may indicate a transitory virus-induced symptom.
4. Visual field changes and neurologic motor or sensory alterations in other locations may indicate multiple sclerosis or diabetes.

Diagnostic Procedures

1. For V2 paresthesia, sinus films, head computed tomography scans, or magnetic resonance images should be obtained to detect antral tumor.
2. For V3 paresthesia, panoramic and periapical films are needed to assess for irregular radiolucencies indicative of metastatic cancer.
3. History of malignancy elsewhere in the organ systems should be evaluated.
4. Fasting blood sugar should be measured to determine the presence of diabetes mellitus.
5. Complete neurologic assessment is necessary for multiple sclerosis, and serologic assessment is undertaken for antimyelin antibodies.
6. Surgical biopsy of sinus or bone should be performed to determine the specific diagnosis when disease is present.

Management

1. For suspected diabetes mellitus or multiple sclerosis, the patient should be referred to an appropriate medical specialist (internist, neurologist).
2. No treatment is necessary for nerve trauma due to third molar surgery. Most resolve spontaneously, with return of sensation.
3. The patient should be referred to a head and neck surgeon for primary tumor or a medical oncologist for metastatic tumors.

Muscle Paresis (Motor Deficits)

Bell's palsy
Neoplasm
Stroke

Significant Findings

1. Localization of paralyzed muscle groups according to nerve distribution is necessary. Paralysis of nerve III, IV, or VI indicates ophthalmoplegia; V, mastication muscles; VII, facial expression (total face—peripheral nerve tracts involved; lower face only—central nervous system tract involvement by tumor or vascular disease); XII, deviated tongue movements.
2. Examination for parotid malignancy (nerve VII) or skull base and parapharyngeal malignancies must be undertaken based on physical signs and imaging.
3. A history of sudden, abrupt nerve VII paralysis is indicative of Bell's palsy.
4. Presence of pain and vesicular eruption of the external ear canal with facial paralysis indicates varicella zoster involvement of nerve VII (Ramsay Hunt syndrome).
5. Hypertensive patients may have a stroke etiology.

Diagnostic Procedures

1. Complete cranial nerve function tests must be conducted.
2. A palpable preauricular or subauricular mass indicates parotid tumor, adenoid cystic carcinoma being the more common type to cause paresis of nerve VII as a result of its neurotropic feature.
3. Evoked potentials of nerve VII can assess the degree of damage.
4. Varicella zoster virus antibody titer can be measured when recurrent viral disease is suspected with cytologic smear of ear vesicles for identification of the virus.
5. Tumor must be ruled out with computed tomography or magnetic resonance imaging.

Management

1. Bell's palsy can be successfully managed with prescription of steroids and vitamin B_{12} injections.
2. Detection of tumor requires biopsy or fine-needle aspiration to determine histologic type. Tumors metastatic to the skull base also encroach upon cranial nerves as they exit their foramina.
3. Stroke patients should be under the care of a general physician or internist.

Oral Therapeutics and Pharmacopeia

Prophylaxis

ENDOCARDITIS PREVENTION

Regimen A, Adults

Rx
> Amoxicillin 500 mg
> Dsp: #9
> Sig: 6 caps 1 hour before procedure; 3 caps 6 hours later

Adults Allergic to Penicillin

Rx
> Erythromycin ethylsuccinate 400 mg
> Dsp: #3
> Sig: 2 tabs 2 hours before procedure; 1 tab 6 hours later

Rx
> Erythromycin stearate 500 mg
> Dsp: #3
> Sig: 2 tabs 2 hours before procedure; 1 tab 6 hours later

Rx
> Erythromycin 250 mg (E-Mycin)
> Dsp: #6
> Sig: 4 tabs 2 hours before procedure; 2 tabs 6 hours later

Note: Enteric coated for individuals with erythromycin gastric sensitivity.

Adults Allergic to Penicillin and Erythromycin

Rx
> Clindamycin 150 mg
> Dsp: #3
> Sig: 2 caps 1 hour before procedure; 1 cap 6 hours later

Regimen B, Adults
Adults at Severe Risk

Rx
> Ampicillin 2 gm
> Gentamicin 1.5 mg/kg
> Sig: IV or IM; not to exceed 80 mg, 1 hour before
>   procedure

Adults With Prosthetic Valves and Who Are Allergic to Penicillin

Rx | Vancomycin 1-g IV drip over 1 hour

Regimen A, Children
Children Under 33 Pounds

Rx | Amoxicillin 250 mg
Dsp: #5
Sig: 3 caps 1 hour before procedure; 2 caps 6 hours later

Children Between 33 and 66 Pounds

Rx | Amoxicillin 250 mg
Dsp: #9
Sig: 6 caps 1 hour before procedure; 3 caps 6 hours later

Children Under 66 Pounds Who Are Allergic to Penicillin

Rx | Erythromycin ethylsuccinate or stearate
Sig: 20-mg/kg initial dose 2 hours before procedure;
10-mg/kg dose 6 hours later

Children Under 66 Pounds Who Are Allergic to Penicillin and Erythromycin

Rx | Clindamycin
Sig: 30-mg/kg initial dose 1 hour before procedure;
15-mg/kg dose 6 hours later

Regimen B, Children at Severe Risk or with Prosthetic Valves.

Rx | Ampicillin 50 mg/kg
Gentamicin 10 mg/kg
Sig: IV or IM 1 hour before procedure
Amoxicillin 25 mg/kg 6 hours later

Odontogenic and Periodontal Infections

In nonallergic patients, penicillin is generally the drug of choice for pulpal and periodontal infections. Culture and sensitivity testing should be performed when abscess, space infection, cellulitis, or osteomyelitis is evident. In this way, the appropriate antibiotic can be selected should the infection fail to resolve.

Certain forms of nonacute periodontitis (juvenile and refractory adult forms) can be treated with tetracyclines and metronidazole.

Rx

> Amoxicillin 500 mg
> Dsp: #40
> Sig: 1 cap every 6 hours for 10 days

Rx

> Amoxicillin 500 mg
> Clavulanate potassium 125 mg
> Dsp: #40
> Sig: 1 tab every 6 hours for 10 days

Rx

> Penicillin V potassium 500 mg
> Dsp: #40
> Sig: 1 cap every 6 hours for 10 days

Rx

> Erythromycin stearate 500 mg or E-Mycin 250 mg
> Dsp: #40
> Sig: 1 cap every 6 hours for 10 days

Rx

> Clindamycin 150 mg
> Dsp: #40
> Sig: 2 caps every 6 hours for 10 days

Rx

> Dicloxacillin 150 mg
> Dsp: #40
> Sig: 2 caps every 6 hours for 10 days

Rx | Cephalexin 250 mg
Dsp: #40
Sig: 1 cap every 6 hours for 10 days

Rx | Tetracycline hydrochloride 250 mg
Dsp: #40
Sig: 1 cap every 6 hours for 10 days

Rx | Metronidazole hydrochloride 250 mg
Dsp: #28
Sig: 1 tab every 6 hours for 7 days

Rx | Metronidazole hydrochloride 250 mg
Dsp: #6
Sig: 3 tabs followed by 3 more tabs 6 hours later

Rx | Chlorhexidine 0.12%
Dsp: Three 1 pt bottles
Sig: rinse twice daily for 30 seconds, expectorate; $\frac{1}{2}$ oz

Candidiasis

Rx | Nystatin ointment
Dsp: 30 g
Sig: apply to corners of mouth (angular cheilitis) or inner surface of denture (denture-associated *Candida*) 4 times daily

Rx | Nystatin pastilles 200,000 U
Dsp: #80
Sig: 2 tabs 4 times a day orally as lozenges

Rx
> Clotrimazole troches 10 mg
> Dsp: #40
> Sig: 1 tab every 6 hours orally as a lozenge

Rx
> Ketoconazole 200 mg
> Dsp: #10
> Sig: 1 tab before bedtime

Rx
> Fluconazole 100 mg
> Dsp: #11
> Sig: 2 tabs initial dose, 1 tab per day thereafter

Viral Infections

HERPES

Rx
> Acyclovir ointment 5%
> Dsp: 15 g
> Sig: Apply to lip 6 times daily

Note: Preferably, the ointment should be applied at the onset of prodromal paresthesia.

Prevention of Recurrent Flare-Ups

Rx
> Acyclovir 800 mg
> Dsp: #9
> Sig: 1 cap twice daily 1 day before dental appointment,
>   then 1 cap each day for 7 days

Long-Term Prophylaxis

Rx
> Acyclovir 800 mg
> Dsp: #30
> Sig: 1 cap daily
> Refill monthly

ACTIVE ORAL HERPES SIMPLEX, CYTOMEGALOVIRUS, HAIRY LEUKOPLAKIA, AND HERPES ZOSTER

Rx

> Acyclovir 800 mg
> Dsp: #20
> Sig: 1 cap twice each day until gone

Odontogenic Pain

MILD PAIN

Rx

> Aspirin 325 mg
> Sig: 2 tabs every 6 hours as needed for pain

Rx

> Ibuprofen 600 mg
> Sig: 1 cap every 4 hours as needed for pain

Rx

> Acetaminophen 325 mg
> Sig: 2 caps every 6 hours as needed for pain

Rx

> Propoxyphene HCl 65 mg/aspirin 389 mg/caffeine 32.4 mg
> (Darvon Compound-65)
> Dsp: #40
> Sig: 1 cap every 4 hours as needed for pain

MODERATE PAIN

Rx

> Aspirin 325 mg with codeine #3 (30 mg)
> Dsp: #40
> Sig: 1 or 2 tabs every 6 hours as needed for pain

Rx

> Aspirin 325 mg with codeine #4 (60 mg)
> Dsp: #40
> Sig: 1 tab every 6 hours as needed for pain

Rx | Acetaminophen 325 mg with codeine #3 (30 mg)
Dsp: #40
Sig: 2 caps every 6 hours as needed for pain

Rx | Acetaminophen 325 mg with codeine #4 (60 mg)
Dsp: #40
Sig: 1 cap every 6 hours as needed for pain

Rx | Ketorolac tromethamine 10 mg (Toradol)
Dsp: #40
Sig: 1 tab every 6 hours as needed for pain

Rx | Oxycodone hydrochloride (Percodan, Percocet)
Dsp: #20
Sig: 1 tab every 4 hours as needed for pain

Rx | Hydrocodone bitartrate 5 mg (Vicodin) or 10 mg (Vicodin
Plus)
Dsp: #20
Sig: 1 tab every 4 hours as needed for pain

Rx | Butalbital 50 mg/aspirin or acetaminophen 325 mg/
caffeine 40 mg (Fiorinal, Fioricet)
Dsp: #40
Sig: 1 or 2 tabs every 4 hours as needed for pain

Note: This regimen is useful for promoting sleep.

SEVERE PAIN

Rx | Meperidine hydrochloride 50 mg (Demerol)
Dsp: #20
Sig: 1 tab every 4 hours as needed for pain

Rx | Hydromorphone hydrochloride 2 mg (Dilaudid)
Dsp: #12
Sig: 1 tab every 4 hours as needed for pain

Note: Both regimens for severe pain are highly addictive.

Nonodontogenic Pain

NEURALGIC AND VASCULAR PAIN SYNDROMES

Rx | Nifedipine 10 mg
Dsp: #60
Sig: 1 cap twice daily

Rx | Diltiazem 60 mg
Dsp: #55
Sig: 1 tab twice daily for 5 days; 1 tab 3 times a day
thereafter

*Note: Both regimens are calcium channel blockers effective in the treatment
of cluster headache and the prevention of midface vascular pain.*

Rx | Ergotamine tartrate with caffeine (Cafergot) suppositories
Dsp: #10
Sig: 1 tab placed rectally at onset of pain attack

*Note: This should not be administered to patients with hypertension or
pregnancy. Ergot causes intestinal side effects. Do not use more than 5 doses
per week.*

Giant Cell Arteritis of Temporal or Facial Artery

Rx | Prednisone 10 mg
Dsp: #30
Sig: 1 tab each day

Trigeminal and Glossopharyngeal Neuralgias

Rx | Carbamazepine 100 mg
Dsp: #40
Sig: 1 tab 2 times a day for 2 days; 1 tab 3 times a day
thereafter

*Note: Dose may be increased up to 800 mg / day. The patient should be
monitored with complete blood counts, since a dose-dependent bone marrow
suppression occurs with carbamazepine.*

ATYPICAL FACIAL PAIN AND BURNING MUCOSA

These are chemically unrelated antidepressants that can be used in
the treatment of facial pain associated with depression. Maintenance

doses may have to be continued for many months. Dosage should be adjusted to levels at which pain symptoms resolve.

Rx Amitriptyline hydrochloride 50 mg
Dsp: #45
Sig: 1 cap each evening for 5 days, then 2 caps each evening for 5 days, then 3 caps each evening before bedtime

Rx Doxepin hydrochloride 25 mg
Dsp: #45
Sig: 1 cap each evening for 5 days, then 2 caps each evening for 5 days, then 4 caps each evening before bedtime

Rx Trazodone hydrochloride 50 mg
Dsp: #70
Sig: 2 tabs each evening for 5 days, then 3 tabs each evening for 5 days, then 3 tabs 3 times daily

Rx Fluoxetine hydrochloride 20 mg
Dsp: #30
Sig: ½ cap daily

Anxiety and Muscle Tension

ANXIOLYTICS

These axiolytics can be used by phobic patients before appointments. Short-term (1- to 2-week) therapy may be useful in facial myalgic pain; longer use may result in dependence.

Rx Diazepam 5 mg
Dsp: #20
Sig: 1 or 2 tabs daily (or 1 hour before office visit)

Rx Lorazepam 1 mg
Dsp: #20
Sig: 1 or 2 tabs daily (or 1 hour before office visit)

Rx

Alprazolam 0.25 mg
Dsp: #20
Sig: 1 tab 3 times daily (or 1 tab 1 hour before office visit)

MUSCLE RELAXANTS

Rx

Chlorzoxazone with acetominophen 500 mg
Dsp: #100
Sig: 2 tabs every 4 hours

Rx

Baclofen 10 mg
Dsp: #60
Sig: ½ tab 3 times daily for 3 days, then 1 tab 3 times daily
for 3 days, then 1½ tabs 3 times daily

Facial Myalgia

Rx

Cyclobenzaprine hydrochloride 10 mg
Dsp: #42
Sig: 1 tab 3 times daily

Note: Short-term use is recommended. This regimen can be prescribed along with nonsteroidal anti-inflammatory drugs.

Soft Tissue Pain From Ulcers, Vesicles, and Erosions

Rx

2% Xylocaine Viscous
Dsp: 4 oz
Sig: 3 drops applied with fingertip to sore areas or placed
on pacifier

Note: This preparation is for infants who are unable to rinse. Since anesthesia of the oropharynx can occur with diminution of the gag reflex, the parents should be instructed to observe child closely while he or she is taking food or liquids after administration of the anesthetic.

Rx | Diphenhydramine hydrochloride (Benadryl) elixer
12.5 mg/tsp 50:50 with Kaopectate
Dsp: 8 oz
Sig: 2 tsp used as a topical rinse and expectorated, as
needed for oral discomfort and pain

Rx | Promethazine (Phenergan) syrup 6.25 mg/tsp 50:50 with
Kaopectate
Dsp: 8 oz
Sig: 2 tsp used as a topical rinse and expectorated, as
needed for oral discomfort and pain

Note: Patient should be told to avoid swallowing and that the medication can cause constipation and drowsiness. Xylocaine 1% can be added to these cocktails for added anesthetic effects. These rinses are palliative and have no therapeutic effects. Allergic reactions to them are extremely rare.

Rx | Chlortetracycline oral suspension (Aureomycin)
250 mg/tsp
Dsp: 8 oz
Sig: 2 tsp used as a topical rinse and expectorated, as
needed for oral discomfort and pain

Note: Tooth discoloration could evolve if this preparation is used chronically and swallowed. This rinse has therapeutic effects for recurrent aphthous ulcers but is of no benefit for other oral ulcerative, vesiculobullous diseases.

Bullous/Desquamative Diseases (Steroids and Immunosuppressants)

TOPICAL

These topical steroids can be used in conjunction with palliative mouth rinses. They are absorbed into the systemic circulation only in minimal amounts. When gingival lesions are prominent, a soft acrylic splint that extends over the attached gingiva can be used to help occlude the topical steroid gel to the mucosal tissues.

Rx | 0.05% Fluocinonide gel (Lidex)
Dsp: 30 g
Sig: applied to oral sores 6 times a day

Rx | 0.05% Clobetasol propionate ointment (Temovate)
Dsp: 30 g
Sig: applied to oral sores 6 times a day

Rx | 0.05% Halobetasol propionate gel (Ultravate)
Dsp: 30 g
Sig: applied to oral sores 6 times a day

Rx | Dexamethasone elixir 0.1 mg/mL (Decadron)
Dsp: 8 oz
Sig: 1 to 2 tsp used as an oral rinse 4 to 6 times a day and
expectorated

SYSTEMIC

Rx | Methylprednisolone (Medrol) Dosepak
Dsp: 1 package
Sig: Use as stated in the instructions.

Rx | Prednisone 10 mg
Dsp: #60
Sig: 4 tabs each day for 10 days, then 3 tabs each day for
3 days, then 2 tabs each day for 3 days, then 1 tab each
day for 3 days

*Note: Many side effects are associated with long-term steroid therapy. The
loading dose gives favorable results for most oral bullous / desquamative
diseases, and as a short-term intervention, steroids have minimal
complications. Use caution in diabetes since steroids raise blood sugar.
Steroids are contraindicated if an active infection is extant.*

Rx | Dapsone 25 mg
Dsp: #30
Sig: 1 tab daily for 3 days, then 2 tabs daily for 3 days,
then 3 tabs daily for 3 days, then 2 tabs twice a day

*Note: Hemolysis is a complication, so hemoglobin, hematocrit, and red cell
counts should be monitored.*

Rx	Azathioprine 50 mg (Imuran) Dsp: #30 Sig: 1 tab daily in conjunction with prednisone

Note: Azathioprine induces bone marrow suppression, so the complete blood cell count should be monitored. Azathioprine with prednisone is indicated in patients who do not respond well to the steroid alone.

Cessation of Smoking and Smokeless Tobacco Use

Rx	Nicotine polacrilex gum 2 mg Dsp: #96 Sig: Tobacco use is stopped, and 10 to 15 sticks are chewed per day for 20 to 30 minutes; after 1 week, the dosage is progressively reduced, by 3 or 4 sticks every 4 days.

Rx	Nicotine transdermal patch 21 mg Dsp: 2, 14 system packages Sig: Tobacco use is stopped, and 1 patch is placed on the hairless skin of the upper body each day.

Then:

Rx	Nicotine transdermal patch 14 mg Dsp: 1, 14 system packages Sig: Tobacco use is stopped, and 1 patch is placed on the hairless skin of the upper body each day.

Then:

Rx	Nicotine transdermal patch 7 mg Dsp: 1, 14 system packages Sig: Tobacco use is stopped, and 1 patch is placed on the hairless skin of the upper body each day.

Miscellaneous Preparations

DRY SOCKET PREVENTION

CAUTION: Do not prescribe for patients with vascular occlusive disease.

> **Rx** Epsilon-aminocaproic acid 500 mg
> Dsp: 14 tabs
> Sig: 8 tabs immediately after or just before extraction,
>   then 2 tabs every 4 hours for 12 hours

HYPERSALIVATION

CAUTION: Do not prescribe for patients with glaucoma, myasthenia gravis, obstructive bowel disease, or obstructive urinary bladder disease.

> **Rx** Propantheline bromide 15 mg
> Dsp: 10 tabs
> Sig: 1 or 2 tabs 1 hour before dental appointment

TOPICAL HEMOSTASIS

Thrombin (thrombogen)

> **Rx** 1000-U vials
> Topical solution can be applied to gauze squares and
>   compressed over bleeding site; it is reconstituted with
>   diluent.

> **Rx** Topical spray tip is available for direct application to area
>   of bleed

XEROSTOMIA

CAUTION: Do not prescribe or prescribe with caution for patients with hypertension, arrhythmia, biliary disease, urolithiasis, or psychosis.

> **Rx** Pilocarpine HCl 5 mg
> Dsp: 100 tabs
> Sig: 1 tab 3 times daily, may increase up to 6 tablets per
>   day after 1 week

Injection Drug Regimens

THROMBIN (THROMBOSTAT): To stop excessive local bleeds in those with coagulation defects.

Rx	5 mg/vial, 10 mg/vial Reconstituted with provided diluent

Note: Use immediately after preparation. Thrombin may cause fatal thrombosis if injected into large vessel.

SODIUM TETRADECYL SULFATE (SOTRADECOL): Sclerosis of labial varices and oral Kaposi's sarcoma.

Rx	3%, 2-ml ampule Aspirated into 1-mL tuberculin syringe, and injected into center and peripheral aspects of vascular lesion as minute amounts (0.02 to 0.05 mL) in multiple foci

Note: For Kaposi's sarcoma, procedure may require 2 or 3 treatments.

VINBLASTINE SULFATE (VELBAN): Treatment of oral Kaposi's sarcoma.

Rx	10 mg/10-mL vial Aspirated into 1-ml tuberculin syringe, and multiple 0.1-mL injections are made into the tumor mass, with the total amount injected dependent on the size of the tumor.

Note: Up to 5 treatments may be necessary.

TRIAMCINOLONE ACETONIDE (KENALOG 40, ARISTOCORT 25 OR 40): Intralesional injection of bullous lesions, noninfectious granulomatous swellings (e.g., cheilitis granulomatosa).

Rx	25- and 40-mg/mL suspension Aspirated into an emptied local anesthetic Carpule or a tuberculin syringe, and multiple injections of 0.05 to 0.1 mL are made into the submucosa or into the bulk tissue or granuloma

Drugs for Medical Emergencies

Many drug emergency kits for the dental office are commercially available.

HYPERSENSITIVITY REACTIONS

Anaphylactic Shock

Injectable **epinephrine 1:1000** (1 mg/mL) in 1-mL ampules; intramuscular or sublingual, 0.3 to 0.5 ml

Immediate Hypersensitivity (IgE-Mediated) Without Airway Shutdown

Injectable **chlorpheniramine (10 mg/mL)** or **diphenhydramine (50 mg/mL)** in 1-mL ampules; intramuscular or sublingual, 1 mL

Immediate or Delayed Hypersensitivity (IgE, T cell)

Hydrocortisone sodium succinate 50 mg/ml (2-mL vial) or **methylprednisolone sodium succinate 40 mg/mL,** (1-mL vial) used as an adjunct with epinephrine or antihistamine; intramuscular, 1 mL

SEIZURES

Diazepam 5 mg/mL (2-mL loaded syringe); intramuscular or sublingual, 1 to 2 mL

SEVERE INTRACTABLE PAIN

Morphine sulfate 10 mg/mL (1-mL vial) or **meperidine 50 mg/ml** (1-mL vial); intramuscular, 1 mL)

NARCOTIC OVERDOSE

Naloxone 0.4 mg/mL (1-mL ampule); intramuscular, 1 mL

ASTHMA

Metaproterenol inhaler for 1 or 2 inhalations
Epinephrine 1:1000 (1 mg/mL) in 1-mL ampules; intramuscular or sublingual 0.3 to 0.5 mL for severe attack
Aminophylline 250 mg in intravenous slow drip, also for severe attack

HYPOTENSIVE SHOCK OR MAJOR SYNCOPE

Aromatic ammonia (Vaporole, 0.3 mL) crushed near nostril
Methoxamine 10 mg/mL (1-mL ampule) or **phenylephrine 10 mg/ mL** (1-mL ampule), for hypotension from drug overdose, postseizure, acute adrenal insufficiency; intramuscular 1 mL

INSULIN (HYPOGLYCEMIC) SHOCK
Oral glucose (any cola, orange juice, or candy bar in conscious patients)

50% Dextrose solution for intravenous administration or **glucagon 1 mg/mL;** intramuscular 1 mL

DIABETIC (HYPERGLYCEMIC) SHOCK

Basic life support administered until medical assistance arrives. Insulin should be titrated only when blood glucose levels can be monitored.

ANGINA PECTORIS

Nitroglycerine tabs 0.3 mg, 1 tab sublingually

ADVANCED CARDIAC LIFE SUPPORT DRUGS

(To be used by trained practitioners)
Sodium bicarbonate 1 mEq/mL (50-mL ampule) for acidosis accompanying cardiopulmonary arrest
Calcium chloride 100 mg/mL (10-mL ampule) to release ventricular arrest
Lidocaine 10 mg/mL (10-mL preloaded syringe) for arrythmia, ventricular prematurities, fibrillation, or tachycardia
Atropine sulfate 0.1 mg/mL (5-ml preloaded syringe) for severe sinus bradycardia with hypotension

PART VI

Precautions and Drug Interactions for Oral Therapeutic Agents

Therapeutic Agents Prescribed in Dental Practice

The drugs that are prescribed for dental and oral diseases are quite limited when one considers the plethora of medications available. In some ways, the fact that dentists use only a small number of prescription drugs is comforting, since remembering the pharmacology of all the drugs that are rarely used is not feasible. This section lists the drugs that are most commonly prescribed in dental practice and enumerates their indications, complications, and interactions with other drugs that the patient may be taking for various medical illnesses.

ANTIBACTERIALS

AMOXICILLIN (Amoxil, Augmentin, Novamoxin, Trimox, Wymox, Polymox, Apo-Amoxi, Clavulin): endocarditis, odontogenic infections

PENICILLIN V (Pen VK, Ledercillin VK, Nadopen V, Novapen V, PVK, V-Cillin K): endocarditis, odontogenic infections

ADVERSE EFFECTS: allergy, discoloration of tongue

CAUTIONS: Prescribe with care or do not use if the patient is allergic, taking birth control pills, or nursing a child.

INTERACTIONS:
1. other antibiotics (chloramphenicol, erythromycin, tetracyclines)—decreased effect of both antibiotics
2. antacids—decreased absorption of antibiotic
3. birth control pills—decreased contraceptive effect
4. beta-blockers—anaphylaxis if allergic reaction occurs
5. calcium—decreased antibiotic effect
6. cimetidine—decreased absorption of antibiotic
7. probenecid—decreased antibiotic effect
8. colestipol—decreased antibiotic effect

ERYTHROMYCIN (Erythrocin, Ilosone, Erycette, E-Mycin, Wyamycin-S): endocarditis, odontogenic infections.

ADVERSE EFFECTS: nausea, diarrhea

CAUTIONS: Prescribe with care or do not use if the patient is allergic, has liver disease, or is nursing a child.

INTERACTIONS
1. other antibiotics (lincomycin, penicillins)—decreased antibiotic effect
2. caffeine—increased caffeine effects
3. warfarin—increased bleeding
4. aminophylline—potentiated bronchodilator and coronary dilator effect

5. theophylline—increased theophylline levels with arrhythmia
6. oxtriphylline—increased oxtriphylline levels with arrhythmia

CLINDAMYCIN (Cleocin): gram-negative anaerobic bacilli, odontogenic infections

ADVERSE EFFECTS: bloating, diarrhea, rare, potentially fatal pseudomembranous colitis that is reversed by vancomycin

CAUTIONS: Prescribe with care or do not use if the patient is allergic or pregnant, or has ulcerative colitis, oral candidiasis, severe renal disease, or severe liver disease.

INTERACTIONS:
1. other antibiotics (chloramphenicol, erythromycin)—decreased clindamycin effect
2. antidiarrheals—decreased antibiotic effect
3. loperamide—worsened clindamycin-induced colitis
4. diphenoxylate—worsened clindamycin-induced colitis
5. muscle-blocking drugs—dangerously increased blocker action

CEPHALEXIN (Keflex, Keftab, Novolexin, Entacef, Ceporex): odontogenic infection for susceptible organisms

ADVERSE EFFECT: diarrhea

CAUTIONS: Prescribe with care or do not use if the patient is allergic or has colitis, oral candidiasis, or severe renal disease. Patients with allergy to penicillin are often allergic to cephalosporins as well.

INTERACTIONS:
1. other antibiotics (chloramphenicol, erythromycin, clindamycin, tetracyclines)—decreased cephalexin effect
2. alcohol—disulfiram effect
3. foods—delayed absorption
4. nonsteroidal anti-inflammatory drugs—peptic ulcer
5. warfarin—increased bleeding tendency
6. probenecid—increased cephalexin effect

TETRACYCLINE (Achromycin, Apo-Tetra, Declomycin, demeclocycline, Terramycin, doxycycline, oxytetracycline, methacycline, minocycline): topical for recurrent aphthous stomatitis, periodontitis

ADVERSE EFFECTS: candidiasis, dark tongue, dental discoloration with long-term use.

CAUTIONS: Prescribe with care or do not use if the patient is allergic or pregnant

INTERACTIONS: None for the topical preparation that is expectorated; with systemic use:
1. food—minerals, milk, and dairy products decrease absorption of tetracycline

2. antacids—decreased absorption
3. penicillin—decreased penicillin effect
4. warfarin—increased bleeding tendency
5. birth control pills—decreased contraceptive effect
6. cholestyramine, colestipol—decreased tetracycline effect
7. digitalis—decreased digitalis effect
8. etretinate—increased toxicity
9. lithium—increased lithium effect

VANCOMYCIN (Vancocin, Lyphocin P, Vancor, Vancoled): endodontogenic infections, rescue from clindamycin colitis

ADVERSE EFFECTS: not significant

CAUTIONS: prescribe with care or do not use if the patient is allergic or has severe kidney disease, or intestinal obstruction.

INTERACTIONS:
1. other antibiotics (injectable bacitracin, injectable amphotericin B, capreomycin, polymyxin, paromycin, aminoglycosides, streptozocin)—hearing loss, kidney damage
2. colestipol, cholestyramine—hearing loss, kidney damage, decreased vancomycin effect
3. cyclosporine—hearing loss, kidney damage

METRONIDAZOLE (Flagyl, Metizole, Metryl, Metronid, Neo-Tric, Protostat, Satric, Trikacide): chronic, refractory periodontitis

ADVERSE EFFECTS: loss of appetite, nausea, diarrhea, unpleasant taste, metallic taste

CAUTIONS: Prescribe with care or do not use if the patient is allergic, in first trimester of pregnancy, breast-feeding, or anemic, or has other hematologic disorders.

INTERACTIONS:
1. alcohol—disulfiram reaction
2. warfarin—increased bleeding
3. disulfiram—adverse symptoms
4. phenobarbital—decreased antibiotic effect
5. phenytoin—decreased antibiotic effect

ANTIFUNGALS

NYSTATIN (Mycostatin, Nilstat, Mycogen, Tri-Statin): oral candidiasis

ADVERSE EFFECT: mild nausea

CAUTION: Do not prescribe if patient is allergic.

INTERACTIONS: none

CLOTRIMAZOLE (MYCLEX): oral candidiasis

ADVERSE EFFECT: mild nausea

CAUTIONS: Prescribe with care or do not use if the patient is allergic, pregnant, breast-feeding, or has severe liver disease.

INTERACTIONS: alcohol, marijuana, cocaine—decreased effect of antifungal agent

KETOCONAZOLE (Nizoral): oral candidiasis

ADVERSE EFFECT: mild nausea

CAUTIONS: Prescribe with care or do not use if the patient is allergic or pregnant, or has achlorhydria or liver disease.

INTERACTIONS:
1. alcohol—liver damage, possible disulfiram reaction
2. tobacco, marijuana, cocaine—decreased antifungal effect
3. antacids—decreased absorption
4. warfarin—increased bleeding
5. anticholinergic agents—decreased absorption of ketoconazole
6. atropine—decreased absorption of ketoconazole
7. belladonna—decreased absorption of ketoconazole
8. cimetidine—decreased absorption of ketoconazole
9. nizatidine—decreased absorption of ketoconazole
10. ranitidine—decreased absorption of ketoconazole
11. scopolamine—decreased absorption of ketoconazole
12. isoniazid—decreased antifungal effect
13. rifampin—decreased antifungal effect
14. hypoglycemics—increased hypoglycemic effect
15. methylprednisolone—increased steroid effect

ANTIVIRALS

ACYCLOVIR (Zovirax): herpes simplex, varicella zoster, hairy leukoplakia

ADVERSE EFFECT: light-headedness

CAUTIONS: Prescribe with care or do not use if the patient is allergic, pregnant, or breast-feeding.

INTERACTIONS:
1. alcohol, marijuana, cocaine—adverse reactions on the central nervous system
2. interferon—neurologic abnormalities
3. methotrexate—neurologic abnormalities
4. antibiotics (amphotericin B, capreomycin, gentamycin, kanamycin, neomycin, polymyxin B, streptomycin, tobramycin, vancomycin, netilmicin)—increased kidney toxicity
5. cyclosporine—increased kidney toxicity
6. probenecid—increased kidney toxicity
7. colistin—increased kidney toxicity
8. zidovudine—increased risk for nerve damage

ANALGESICS

ASPIRIN (many nonprescription brand names and formulations): mild pain

ADVERSE EFFECTS: nausea, tinnitus, indigestion

CAUTIONS: Prescribe with care or do not use if the patient is allergic, on sodium restriction, pregnant, breast-feeding, or has a peptic or duodenal ulcer, a bleeding disorder or chronic liver disease. Children may develop Reye's syndrome.

INTERACTIONS:
1. alcohol—stomach irritation
2. acebutolol—decreased antihypertensive effect
3. carteolol—decreased antihypertensive effect
4. acetylcholinesterase inhibitors—decreased angiotensin-converting enzyme inhibitor effect
5. allopurinol—decreased allopurinol effect
6. antacids—decreased aspirin effect
7. warfarin—increased bleeding
8. indomethacin—risk of stomach ulcer or bleeding
9. diclofenac—risk of stomach ulcer or bleeding
10. steroids—risk of stomach ulcer or bleeding, increased cortisone effect
11. gold—kidney damage
12. furosemide—aspirin toxicity
13. hypoglycemics—accentuated hypoglycemic effect

ACETAMINOPHEN (many nonprescription brand names and formulations): mild pain

ADVERSE EFFECTS: mild nausea, vomiting, fatigue, jaundice, indigestion

CAUTIONS: Prescribe with care or do not use if the patient is allergic, pregnant, breast-feeding, or has a peptic ulcer, a bleeding disorder, or chronic liver disease.

INTERACTIONS:
1. alcohol—stomach irritation, bleeding
2. antacids—decreased drug effect
3. warfarin—increased bleeding tendency
4. salicylates—toxicity
5. barbiturates—liver toxicity
6. carbamazepine—liver toxicity
7. steroids—stomach ulcers or bleeding, increased cortisone effect
8. furosemide—toxicity
9. hypoglycemics—accentuated hypoglycemic effect

IBUPROFEN (Advil, Motrin, Nuprin): mild pain

ADVERSE EFFECTS: mild nausea, dizziness, headache

CAUTIONS: Prescribe with care or do not use if the patient is allergic or breast-feeding, or has a peptic ulcer, colitis, a bleeding disorder, asthma, or chronic liver disease.

INTERACTIONS:
1. antacids—reduced pain relief
2. warfarin—increased bleeding tendency
3. aspirin—stomach ulcer
4. beta-blockers—decreased antihypertensive effect
5. carteolol—decreased antihypertensive effect
6. cephalosporins—increased bleeding
7. steroids—stomach ulcer
8. diuretics—decreased diuresis
9. gold—kidney toxicity

CODEINE (many formulations with aspirin, acetaminophen, and propoxyphene, such as ASA, Empirin, Tylenol, and Darvon): moderate pain

ADVERSE EFFECTS: nausea, constipation, dry mouth, headache

CAUTIONS: Prescribe with care or do not use if the patient is allergic, pregnant, breast-feeding, or driving.

INTERACTIONS: See other listings if formulated.
1. alcohol, marijuana, cocaine—increased intoxication
2. analgesics—increased effect
3. warfarin—increased bleeding
4. antidepressants—increased sedation
5. antihistamines—increased sedation
6. carteolol—dangerous sedation
7. sedatives, hypnotics, anxiolytics—increased sedation
8. selegiline—severe toxicity, coma, seizure
9. monoamine oxidase inhibitors—severe toxicity, death
10. phenothiazine—increased phenothiazine effect
11. zidovudine—increased zidovudine toxicity

HYDROCODONE (formulated with other analgesics: Vicodin, Lorcet, Lortab, Hydrodan, S-T Forte): moderate pain

ADVERSE EFFECTS: nausea, constipation, dry mouth, headache

CAUTIONS: Prescribe with care or do not use if the patient is allergic, pregnant, breast-feeding, or driving, or has respiratory disease or an acute head injury.

INTERACTIONS: See other listings if formulated.
1. alcohol, marijuana, cocaine—increased intoxication
2. analgesics—increased effect
3. warfarin—increased bleeding
4. antidepressants—increased sedation
5. antihistamines—increased sedation
6. carteolol—dangerous sedation
7. sedatives, hypnotics, anxiolytics—increased sedation
8. selegiline—severe toxicity, coma, seizures
9. monoamine oxidase inhibitors—severe toxicity, death
10. phenothiazine—increased phenothiazine effect
11. zidovudine—increased zidovudine toxicity

OXYCODONE (formulated with other analgesics; Percodan, Percocet, Roxicet, Tylox): moderate pain

ADVERSE EFFECTS: nausea, constipation, gastrointestinal cramping, dry mouth, headache

CAUTIONS: Prescribe with care or do not use if the patient is allergic, pregnant, breast-feeding, or driving, or has respiratory disease, or an acute head injury.

INTERACTIONS: See other listings if formulated.
1. alcohol, marijuana, cocaine—increased intoxication
2. analgesics—increased effect
3. warfarin—increased bleeding
4. antidepressants—increased sedation
5. antihistamines—increased sedation
6. carteolol—dangerous sedation
7. sedatives, hypnotics, anxiolytics—increased sedation
8. selegiline—severe toxicity, coma, seizures
9. monoamine oxidase inhibitors—severe toxicity, death
10. phenothiazine—increased phenothiazine effect
11. zidovudine—increased zidovudine toxicity

MEPERIDINE (Demerol, Mepergan): moderate pain

ADVERSE EFFECTS: nausea, constipation, gastrointestinal cramping, dry mouth, headache

CAUTIONS: Prescribe with care or do not use if the patient is allergic, pregnant, breast-feeding, or driving, or has respiratory disease, atrial flutter, a seizure disorder, an acute head injury, or severe liver or renal disease.

INTERACTIONS: See other listings if formulated.
1. alcohol, marijuana, cocaine—increased intoxication
2. analgesics—increased effect
3. warfarin—increased bleeding
4. antidepressants—increased sedation
5. antihistamines—increased sedation
6. carteolol—dangerous sedation
7. sedatives, hypnotics, anxiolytics—increased sedation
8. selegiline—severe toxicity, coma, seizures
9. monoamine oxidase inhibitors—severe toxicity, death
10. phenothiazine—increased phenothiazine effect
11. zidovudine—increased zidovudine toxicity

HYDROMORPHONE HYDROCHLORIDE (Dilaudid): severe pain

ADVERSE EFFECTS: nausea, constipation, gastrointestinal cramping, dry mouth, headache, fainting, orthostatic hypotension

CAUTIONS: Prescribe with care or do not use if the patient is allergic, pregnant, breast-feeding, or driving, or has respiratory disease or an acute head injury.

INTERACTIONS
1. alcohol, marijuana, cocaine—increased intoxication
2. analgesics—increased effect
3. warfarin—increased bleeding
4. antidepressants—increased sedation
5. antihistamines—increased sedation
6. carteolol—dangerous sedation
7. sedatives, hypnotics, anxiolytics—increased sedation
8. selegiline—severe toxicity, coma, seizures
9. monoamine oxidase inhibitors—severe toxicity, death
10. phenothiazine—increased phenothiazine effect
11. zidovudine—increased zidovudine toxicity

CARBAMAZEPINE (Tegretol, Epitol, Maepine, Novocarbamaz, Apo-Carbamazepine): trigeminal neuralgia

ADVERSE EFFECTS: aplastic anemia occurs at higher dosages and therefore CBC and platelet monitoring is essential; erythema multiforme, blurred vision, confusion

CAUTIONS: Prescribe with care or do not use if the patient is allergic or breast-feeding, has vascular occlusive disease or blood dyscrasia.

INTERACTIONS:
1. warfarin—decreased anticoagulant effect
2. hydantoin—decreased effect of both drugs
3. tricyclics, antidepressants, fluoxetine, guanfacine—psychotic or depressive symptoms
4. steroids—decreased steroid effect
5. contraceptives—reduced contraceptive effect
6. digitalis—decreased heart rate
7. erythromycin—increased carbamazepine effect
8. doxycycline—decreased antibiotic effect
9. monoamine oxidase inhibitors—dangerous toxicity

ANTI-INFLAMMATORY AGENTS: STEROIDS AND SULFA DRUGS

TRIAMCINOLONE (Amcort, Aristocort, Kenocort, Cinalone, Kenalog): oral ulcerative or bullous disease

ADVERSE EFFECTS: More nausea, delayed wound healing, increased susceptibility to infection, growth retardation, constipation and diarrhea, mood swings, osteoporosis, edema, facial swelling, increased blood sugar

CAUTIONS: Prescribe with care or do not use if the patient is pregnant or has an active infection, brittle diabetes, osteoporosis, glaucoma, colitis, peptic ulcer, or liver disease.

INTERACTIONS:
1. amphotericin B—depletion of potassium
2. warfarin—decreased anticoagulant effect

3. hydantoin—decreased steroid effect
4. hypoglycemics—decreased antiglycemic effect
5. aspirin—increased steroid activity
6. barbiturates—increased sedation
7. chloral hydrate—decreased steroid effect
8. cholestyramine, colestipol—decreased steroid absorption
9. contraceptives—increased steroid effect
10. digitalis—dangerous potassium depletion
11. thiazides—potassium depletion
12. estrogens—increased steroid effect
13. anticholinergics—possible glaucoma

FLUOCINONIDE (Lidex): oral ulcerative or bullous disease (all preparations are topical)

ADVERSE EFFECTS: None. Appreciable blood levels after short-term oral administration are not encountered.

CAUTION: Prescribe with care or do not use if the patient is pregnant. (Effects of topical agents are not well known.) Long-term use may predispose to oral candidiasis.

INTERACTIONS:
1. Topical antibiotics—decreased antibiotic effect
2. Topical antifungal agents—decreased antimycotic effect

CLOBETASOL (Temovate): oral ulcerative or bullous diseases (all preparations are topical)

ADVERSE EFFECTS: None. Blood levels after short-term oral administration are minimal.

CAUTION: Prescribe with care or do not use if the patient is pregnant. (Effects of topical agents are not well known.) Long-term use may predispose to oral candidiasis.

INTERACTIONS:
1. topical antibiotics—decreased antibiotic effect
2. topical antifungals—decreased antimycotic effect

DEXAMETHASONE (Decadron, Hexadrol): oral suspension topical rinse for ulcerative or bullous diseases

ADVERSE EFFECTS: As an expectorated rinse, none. Appreciable blood levels after short-term oral administration are not seen. If swallowed after rinsing, the same adverse effects listed for systemic steroids may ensue.

CAUTIONS: Prescribe with care or do not use if the patient is pregnant. (Effects of topical agents are not well known.) If swallowed, same cautions apply as with systemic steroids. Long-term use may predispose to oral candidiasis.

INTERACTIONS:
1. topical antibiotics—decreased antibiotic effect
2. topical antifungals—decreased antimycotic effect

3. if swallowed, see triamcinolone or prednisone for listing of similar interactions

PREDNISONE (Deltasone, Prednicen-M, Sterapred): systemic use for severe oral ulcerative or bullous disease

ADVERSE EFFECTS: nausea, delayed wound healing, increased susceptibility to infection, growth retardation, constipation and diarrhea, mood swings, osteoporosis, edema, facial swelling, increased blood sugar

CAUTIONS: Prescribe with care or do not use if the patient is pregnant or has an active infection, brittle diabetes, osteoporosis, glaucoma, colitis, peptic ulcer, or liver disease. Oral candidiasis may occur with prolonged use.

INTERACTIONS:
1. amphotericin B—depletion of potassium
2. warfarin—decreased anticoagulant effect
3. hydantoin—decreased steroid effect
4. hypoglycemics—decreased antiglycemic effect
5. aspirin—increased steroid activity, increased peptic ulcer risk
6. barbiturates—increased sedation
7. chloral hydrate—decreased steroid effect
8. cholestyramine, colestipol—decreased steroid absorption
9. contraceptives—increased steroid effect
10. digitalis—dangerous potassium depletion
11. thiazides—potassium depletion
12. estrogens—increased steroid effect
13. anticholinergics—possible glaucoma
14. furosemide—potassium depletion
15. indapamide—dangerous potassium depletion
16. nonsteroidal anti-inflammatory drugs—increased peptic ulcer risk
17. rifampin—decreased steroid effect
18. phenobarbital—decreased steroid effect
19. theophylline—increased theophylline effect
20. insulin—decreased insulin effect

METHYLPREDNISOLONE (Medrol, Depo-Predate): oral ulcerative or bullous diseases

ADVERSE EFFECTS: nausea, delayed wound healing, increased susceptibility to infection, growth retardation, constipation and diarrhea, mood swings, osteoporosis, edema, facial swelling, increased blood sugar

CAUTIONS: Prescribe with care or do not use if the patient is pregnant or has an active infection, brittle diabetes, osteoporosis, glaucoma, colitis, peptic ulcer, or liver disease.

INTERACTIONS: same as for prednisone

DAPSONE 4-4' diaminodiphenylsulfone): mucous membrane pemphigoid

ADVERSE EFFECTS: dose-dependent methemoglobinemia, pancytopenia, agranulocytosis (requires hemogram monitoring), toxic hepatitis (requires liver function monitoring)

CAUTIONS: Prescribe with care or do not use if the patient is pregnant, breast-feeding, or allergic to any sulfa-containing drugs, thiazide diuretics, or furosemide, or has glucose-6-phosphate deficiency anemia, methemoglobinemia.

INTERACTIONS:
1. methotrexate—agranulocytosis, anemia
2. pyrimethamine—agranulocytosis, anemia
3. probenecid—increased dapsone toxicity
4. rifampin—lowered dapsone blood levels
5. trimethoprim—increased hematologic complications

AZATHIOPRINE (Imuran): severe oral ulcerative or bullous disease

ADVERSE EFFECTS: low blood count, susceptibility to infection, fever, loss of appetite, hepatotoxicity, thrombocytopenia

CAUTIONS: Prescribe with care or do not use if the patient is pregnant or breast-feeding, or has a bleeding diathesis, gout, liver disease, or hematologic disease (anemia, leukemia, neutropenia, thrombocytopenia).

INTERACTIONS:
1. allopurinol—markedly increased azathioprine activity
2. other immunosuppressants—increased infection susceptibility
3. aspirin—increased bleeding

ANXIOLYTICS

BENZODIAZEPINES (diazepam, lorazepam, temazepam, flurazepam, Valium, Ativan, Dalmane, Klonopin, Xanax): preoperative sedation in anxious patients, muscle relaxation in craniofacial and cervical myalgia

ADVERSE EFFECTS: drowsiness, dizziness, hallucinations, behavioral changes, depression, constipation, diarrhea

CAUTIONS: Prescribe with care or do not use if the patient is allergic, or recovering from drug abuse, or has glaucoma, diabetes, epilepsy, porphyria, or myasthenia gravis.

INTERACTIONS:
1. anticonvulsants—alterations in seizure severity
2. antidepressants—increased sedation
3. antihypertensives—significant hypotensive effect
4. clozapine—severe central nervous system toxicity
5. contraceptives—increased sedation
6. disulfiram—increased sedation
7. antibiotics (erythromycin, ketoconazole)—increased sedation

8. L-dopa—decreased levodopa effect
9. monoamine oxidase inhibitors—severe side effects, convulsions
10. narcotics—increased sedation
11. tranquilizers—increased sedation
12. nizatidine—toxic effect of benzodiazapine
13. probenecid—increased sedation
14. zidovudine—bone marrow toxicity

MUSCLE RELAXANTS

BACLOFEN (Lioresal): muscle relaxation for craniofacial and cervical myalgia

ADVERSE EFFECTS: dizziness, confusion, nausea, headache, rash, muscle weakness, slurred speech, impotence

CAUTIONS: Prescribe with care or do not use if the patient is allergic or suffers from cerebral palsy, recent stroke, or myocardial infarction, or if surgery with anesthesia is planned.

INTERACTIONS
1. anesthetics (general)—hypotension, sedation
2. central nervous system depressants—increased sedation
3. clozapine—central nervous system toxicity
4. ethinamate—prolonged sleep
5. fluoxetine—increased depressant effects
6. insulin—altered hypoglycemic effects
7. methyprylon—dangerously increased sedation
8. nabilone—central nervous system depression

CHLORZOXAZONE (Algisin, Flextra, Lobac, Parafon Forte, DSC, Paraforte, Skelex, Mus-Lax, Spasgesic: muscle relaxation for craniofacial and cervical myalgia

ADVERSE EFFECTS: drowsiness, dizziness, dry mouth, dysgeusia, blurred vision, tachycardia, insomnia

CAUTIONS: Prescribe with care or do not use if the patient is allergic or pregnant, or has congestive heart failure, glaucoma, or prostatitis.

INTERACTIONS:
1. alcohol—central nervous system depression
2. anticholinergics—increased anticholinergic effect
3. antidepressants—increased sedation
4. antihistamines—increased antihistaminic effect and sedation
5. barbiturates—increased sedation
6. clonidine—decreased antihypertensive effect
7. clozapine—central nervous system toxicity
8. guanethidine—decreased antihypertensive effect
9. monoamine oxidase inhibitors—severe toxicity, convulsions
10. methyldopa—increased dopa effect
11. narcotics—increased sedation

12. analgesics—increased analgesic effect
13. procainamide—increased arrhythmia
14. quinidine—increased arrhythmia
15. sedatives—increased sedation
16. tranquilizers—increased sedation

CYCLOBENZAPRINE (Flexeril): muscle relaxation for craniofacial and cervical myalgia

ADVERSE EFFECTS: drowsiness, dizziness, dry mouth, dysgeusia, blurred vision, tachycardia, insomnia

CAUTIONS: Prescribe with care or do not use if the patient is allergic or pregnant, or has congestive heart failure, glaucoma, or prostatitis.

INTERACTIONS:
1. alcohol—central nervous system depression
2. anticholinergics—increased anticholinergic effect
3. antidepressants—increased sedation
4. antihistamines—increased antihistaminic effect
5. barbiturates—increased sedation
6. clonidine—decreased antihypertensive effect
7. guanethidine—decreased antihypertensive effect
8. monoamine oxidase inhibitors—severe toxicity, convulsions
9. methyldopa—increased dopa effect
10. narcotics—increased sedation
11. analgesics—increased analgesic effect
12. procainamide—increased arrhythmia
13. quinidine—increased arrhythmia
14. sedatives—increased sedation
15. tranquilizers—increased sedation

ANTIDEPRESSANTS

TRICYCLICS, TETRACYCLICS (amitriptyline, doxepin, Elavil, imipramine, Sinequan, Tofranil): burning mouth syndrome, atypical facial pain and odontalgia

ADVERSE EFFECTS: tremors, headache, fatigue, morning awakening drowsiness, dry mouth, insomnia, indigestion, decreased sex drive, unusual dreams, muscle pain

CAUTIONS: Do not prescribe if the patient has a history of allergy. Do not prescribe for patients with glaucoma and women who are breast feeding. Use caution in patients with hypertension, hyperthyroidism, asthma, inflammatory bowel disease, or prostatic hypertrophy.

INTERACTIONS:
1. alcohol—exaggerated intoxication
2. anticoagulants—hemorrhagic tendency
3. anticholinergics—increased anticholinergic effect, dryness
4. antihistamines—increased antihistaminic effect, dryness
5. barbiturates—increased sedation and depression

   6. benzodiazepines—accentuated sedation
   7. cocaine—cardiac arrhythmia
   8. sedative/hypnotic narcotics—increased sedation

FLUOXETINE (Prozac): burning mouth syndrome, atypical facial pain and odontalgia

ADVERSE EFFECTS: headache, drowsiness, nervousness, insomnia, diarrhea, decreased sex drive, altered dreams

CAUTIONS: Do not prescribe or prescribe with care if the patient has severe renal or liver disease.

INTERACTIONS:
   1. alcohol—accentuated intoxication
   2. anticoagulants—hypertension, convulsions
   3. cocaine—decreased antidepressant effects
   4. digitalis—hypertension, convulsions
   5. monoamine oxidase inhibitors—hypertension, convulsions
   6. tryptophan—nervousness, agitation
   7. sedative/hypnotic narcotics—increased sedation

SEDATIVE-HYPNOTICS

CHLORAL HYDRATE (Aquachloral, Noctec, Novochlorhydrate): preoperative pediatric sedation

ADVERSE EFFECTS: nausea, drowsiness, dizziness, diarrhea, leukopenia, habit-forming

CAUTIONS: Prescribe with care or do not use if the patient is allergic to chloral hydrate or tartrazine dyes or is pregnant, or has liver or kidney disease.

INTERACTIONS:
   1. anticoagulants—increased bleeding
   2. antidepressants—increased sedation
   3. antihistamines—increased sedation
   4. clozapine—central nervous system toxicity
   5. monoamine oxidase inhibitors—increased sedation
   6. methyprylon—marked sedation
   7. narcotics—increased sedation
   8. phenothiazines—increased sedation
   9. sedatives—increased sedation
   10. tranquilizers—increased sedation

BARBITURATES (Alurate, Butisol, Nembutal): intermediate acting for preoperative sedation in adults

ADVERSE EFFECTS: dizziness, drowsiness, hangover, depression, confusion, diarrhea, nausea

CAUTIONS: Prescribe with care or do not use if the patient is pregnant or allergic, or has porphyria, asthma, anemia, epilepsy, liver disease, or renal disease.

INTERACTIONS:
1. anticoagulants—decreased anticoagulation effect
2. anticonvulsants—altered seizures
3. antidepressants—increased sedation, counteracted antidepressant effect
4. antihistamines—marked sedation
5. aspirin—decreased analgesia
6. beta-blockers—decreased β-adrenergic effect
7. carbamazepine—decreased pain relief in trigeminal neuralgia
8. carteolol—increased sedation
9. clozapine—central nervous system toxicity
10. contraceptives—decreased contraceptive effect
11. divalproex—marked sedation
12. doxycycline—decreased antimicrobial effect
13. griseofulvin—decreased antifungal effect
14. hypoglycemics—increased sedation
15. monoamine oxidase inhibitors—increased sedation
16. narcotics—increased sedation
17. sedatives—marked sedation

ANTIHISTAMINES

DIPHENHYDRAMINE (Allerdryl, Benadryl): to reverse a type I allergic reaction (e.g., penicillin reaction, allergic stomatitis)

ADVERSE EFFECTS: drowsiness, dizziness, dry mouth or airway, loss of appetite, bleeding tendency

CAUTIONS: Prescribe with care or do not use if the patient has glaucoma, prostatic hypertrophy, or peptic ulcer, or is breast-feeding.

INTERACTIONS:
1. anticholinergics—increased anticholinergic effect
2. anticoagulants—decreased antihistaminic effect
3. antidepressants—increased sedation
4. carteolol—decreased antihistaminic effect
5. clozapine—central nervous system toxicity
6. sedative/hypnotics—excess sedation
7. monoamine oxidase inhibitors—increased antihistaminic effect
8. molindone—increased sedation
9. nabilone—central nervous system depression
10. tranquilizers, anxiolytics—increased sedation

PROMETHAZINE (Mepergan, Phenergan): to reverse a type I allergic reaction (e.g., penicillin reaction, allergic stomatitis)

ADVERSE EFFECTS: drowsiness, dizziness, dry mouth or airway, loss of appetite, bleeding tendency

CAUTIONS: Prescribe with care or do not use if the patient has glaucoma, prostatic hypertrophy, or peptic ulcer, or is breast-feeding.

INTERACTIONS:
1. anticholinergics—increased anticholinergic effect
2. anticoagulants—decreased antihistaminic effect
3. antidepressants—increased sedation
4. carteolol—decreased antihistaminic effect
5. clozapine—central nervous system toxicity
6. sedative/hypnotics—excess sedation
7. monoamine oxidase inhibitors—increased antihistaminic effect
8. molindone—increased sedation
9. nabilone—central nervous system depression
10. tranquilizers, anxiolytics—increased sedation

ANTINEOPLASTICS

5% FLUOROURACIL CREAM (Fluoroplex, Efudex): actinic cheilitis, actinic keratosis

ADVERSE EFFECTS: pain and burning of treated skin, burning of eyes, local hyperpigmentation

CAUTIONS: Do not prescribe if the patient is allergic. Do not use with other creams, ointments, or lotions.

INTERACTIONS: for topical application, none.

SIALOGOGUES

PILOCARPINE HYDROCHLORIDE (Salagen)

ADVERSE EFFECTS: hypertension, hypotension, bradycardia, tachycardia, sweating, biliary spasm

CAUTIONS: Do not prescribe if patient is allergic. Prescribe with caution if patient is hypertensive or has cardiovascular disease, arrhythmia, biliary disease, urolithiasis, or psychosis.

INTERACTIONS:
Anticholinergics—decreases anticholinergic effects
Beta-blockers—increases risk for arrhythmia
Parasympathomimetics—increases effect

MOUTH RINSE PREPARATIONS

ANTIHISTAMINES (promethazine and diphenhydramine syrup or elixir, 50/50 Kaopectate): palliative mouth rinse for oral ulcers and erosions

ADVERSE EFFECTS: minimal if not swallowed. If swallowed, same as systemically administered antihistamines.

CAUTIONS: None.

INTERACTIONS: Minimal if not swallowed. If swallowed, same as systemically administered antihistamines. Antihistaminic mouth rinses may be formulated with steroids and anesthetics.

STEROIDAL—See dexamethasone

ANESTHETIC: 2% Lidocaine viscous (Xylocaine Viscous): sore mouth, oral ulcerations, oral erosions

ADVERSE EFFECTS: Excessive use predisposes to dental caries. Lidocaine may inhibit gag reflex, resulting in food aspiration in infants or young children.

CAUTIONS: Prescribe with care or do not use if the patient has a history of allergy to anesthetics.

INTERACTIONS: reduces effects of sulfa antibiotics

CHLORHEXIDINE GLUCONATE (Peridex): periodontal disease, gingivitis, candidiasis, aphthous ulcers

ADVERSE EFFECTS: brown staining of teeth and dorsum of tongue, dysgeusia

CAUTIONS: Prescribe with care or do not use if the patient is allergic.

INTERACTIONS: none known

TETRACYCLINE ORAL SUSPENSION (Aureomycin): recurrent aphthous stomatitis

ADVERSE EFFECTS: Tongue pigmentation. Expectoration of rinse should not be accompanied by other intestinal problems usually associated with swallowing tetracycline.

CAUTIONS: Prescribe with care or do not use if the patient is allergic.

INTERACTIONS: There are many drug interactions if ingested; as a rinse that is expectorated, none are anticipated.

DRUGS ADMINISTERED IN THE OPERATORY

LOCAL ANESTHETICS

2% LIDOCAINE (Xylocaine, Alphacaine, Lignospan, Octocaine): formulated with 1:50,000, 1:100,000, and 1:200,000 epinephrine for dental and oral surgery

ADVERSE EFFECTS: Oral mucosal lacerations secondary to lip, cheek, or tongue biting while numb are common. Most adverse effects occur when the drug is injected intravascularly or too many cartridges are given, and include increased heart rate, elevated blood pressure, increased respiratory rate, nervousness, blurred vision followed by central nervous system depression, seizures, and shock.

CAUTIONS: Administer with care or do not use if the patient has a history of allergic reaction, although most allergies to injection anesthetics are related to the paraben preservatives in the cartridge. Maximum adult levels of administration at a given appointment are 300 mg (8.3 cartridges) when no vasoconstrictor is added. With epinephrine, 500 mg (13.8 cartridges) constitutes the maximum adult dose. When using a vasoconstrictor, care should be taken in patients with hypertension or glaucoma. In severely hypertensive subjects (i.e., diastolic pressure above 110 mm Hg), it is advisable to avoid a vasoconstrictor. If diastolic pressure is below 110, a vasoconstrictor is advisable to maintain deep anesthesia and to avoid loss of pain control, which may stimulate release of endogenous catecholamines. An aspiration syringe should be used, and the anesthetic should not be injected intravascularly. Extreme caution should be taken with patients who have known pseudocholinesterase deficiency (an enzyme that catabolizes procaine and its congeners).

INTERACTIONS:
1. alcohol—central nervous system and respiratory depression
2. antidepressants—central nervous system and respiratory depression
3. antiarrhythmic drugs—cardiac depression
4. antimyasthenic agents—antagonized antimyasthenic effects
5. beta-blockers—prolonged anesthetic effects

VASOCONSTRICTOR INTERACTIONS:
1. inhalation anesthetics—increased risk for arrhythmia
2. beta-blockers—hypertension
3. phenothiazines—hypotension
4. tricyclic antidepressants—tachycardia, systolic hypertension

2% OR 3% MEPIVACAINE (Polocaine, Carbocaine, Arestocaine, Isocaine, Scandonest) formulated without vasoconstrictor (3%) and with vasoconstrictor (2%, 1:20,000 levonordefrin) for dental and oral surgery.

ADVERSE EFFECTS: Oral mucosal lacerations secondary to lip, cheek, or tongue biting while numb are common. Most adverse effects occur when the drug is injected intravascularly or too many cartridges are given, and include increased heart rate, elevated blood pressure, increased respiratory rate, nervousness, blurred vision followed by central nervous system depression, seizures, and shock.

CAUTIONS: Administer with care or do not use if the patient has a history of allergic reactions, although most allergies to injection anesthetics are related to the paraben preservatives in the cartridge. Maximum adult level of administration, with or without vasoconstrictor, at a given appointment is 400 mg (8.5 cartridges). When employing a vasoconstrictor, care should be taken in patients with hypertension or glaucoma. In severely hypertensive subjects (i.e., diastolic pressure above 110 mm Hg), it is advisable to avoid a vasoconstrictor. If diastolic pressure is below 110, a vasoconstrictor is advisable to maintain deep anesthesia and to avoid loss of pain control, which may stimulate release of endogenous catecholamines. An aspiration syringe should be used, and the anesthetic should not be injected intravascularly.

Extreme caution should be taken with patients who have known pseu-docholinesterase deficiency (an enzyme that catabolizes procaine and its congeners).

INTERACTIONS:
1. alcohol—central nervous system and respiratory depression
2. antidepressants—central nervous system and respiratory depression
3. antiarrhythmic drugs—cardiac depression
4. antimyasthenic drugs—antagonized antimyasthenic effects
5. beta-blockers—prolonged anesthetic effects

VASOCONSTRICTOR INTERACTIONS:
1. inhalation anesthetics—increased risk for arrhythmia
2. beta-blockers—hypertension
3. phenothiazines—hypotension
4. tricyclic antidepressants—tachycardia, systolic hypertension

4% PRILOCAINE (Citanest): formulated without vasoconstrictor for dental and oral surgery

ADVERSE EFFECTS: Oral mucosal lacerations secondary to lip, cheek, or tongue biting while numb are common. Most adverse effects occur when the drug is injected intravascularly or too many cartridges are given, and include increased heart rate, elevated blood pressure, increased respiratory rate, nervousness, blurred vision followed by central nervous system depression, seizures, and shock.

CAUTIONS: Prescribe with care or do not use if the patient has a history of allergic reactions, although most allergies to injection anesthetics are related to the paraben preservatives in the cartridge. Maximum adult levels of administration for a given appointment are 600 mg (8.3 cartridges). In hereditary methemoglobinemia, prilocaine is hydro-lyzed to otoluidine, a metabolite that oxidizes hemoglobin to methemo-globin. High blood levels can be dangerous, so another local anesthetic should be selected. Extreme caution should be taken with patients who have known pseudocholinesterase deficiency (an enzyme that catabolizes procaine and its congeners).

INTERACTIONS:
1. alcohol—central nervous system and respiratory depression
2. antidepressants—central nervous system and respiratory depression
3. antiarrhythmic drugs—cardiac depression
4. antimyasthenic drugs—antagonize antimyasthenic effects
5. beta-blockers—prolonged anesthetic effects

0.5% BUPIVACAINE (Marcaine): formulated with 1:200,000 epinephrine for prolonged local anesthesia for dental and oral surgery, local trigger point injections for myalgia

ADVERSE EFFECTS: Oral mucosal lacerations secondary to lip, cheek, or tongue biting while numb are common. Most adverse effects occur when the drug is injected intravascularly or too many cartridges are given, and include increased heart rate, elevated blood pressure, increased respiratory rate, nervousness, blurred vision followed by central nervous system depression, seizures, and shock.

CAUTIONS: Prescribe with care or do not use if the patient has a history of allergic reactions, although most allergies to injection anesthetics are related to the paraben preservatives in the cartridge. When using a vasoconstrictor, care should be taken in patients with hypertension or glaucoma. Maximum adult dose with vasoconstrictor is 90 mg (10 cartridges). In severely hypertensive subjects (i.e., diastolic pressure above 110 mm Hg), it is advisable to avoid anesthetics with vasoconstrictors. If diastolic pressure is below 110, a vasoconstrictor is advisable to maintain deep anesthesia and to avoid endogenous catecholamine release as a consequence of loss of pain control. An aspiration syringe should be used, and the anesthetic should not be injected intravascularly. Extreme caution should be taken with patients who have known pseudocholinesterase deficiency (an enzyme that catabolizes procaine and its congeners).

INTERACTIONS:
1. alcohol—central nervous system and respiratory depression
2. antidepressants—central nervous system and respiratory depression
3. antiarrhythmic drugs—cardiac depression
4. antimyasthenic drugs—antagonize antimyasthenic effects
5. beta-blockers—prolonged anesthetic effects

VASOCONSTRICTOR INTERACTIONS:
1. inhalation anesthetics—increased risk for arrhythmia
2. beta-blockers—hypertension
3. phenothiazines—hypotension
4. tricyclic antidepressants—tachycardia, systolic hypertension

1.5% ETIDOCAINE (Duranest): formulated with 1:200,000 epinephrine for prolonged local anesthesia for dental and oral surgery, local trigger point injections for myalgia

ADVERSE EFFECTS: Oral mucosal lacerations secondary to lip, cheek, or tongue biting while numb are common. Most adverse effects occur when the drug is injected intravascularly or too many cartridges are given and include increased heart rate, elevated blood pressure, increased respiratory rate, nervousness, blurred vision followed by central nervous system depression, seizures, and shock.

CAUTIONS: Prescribe with care or do not use if the patient has a history of allergic reactions, although most allergies to injection anesthetics are related to the paraben preservatives in the cartridge. When using a vasoconstrictor, care should be taken in patients with hypertension or glaucoma. Maximum adult dose with vasoconstrictor is 400 mg (14.7 cartridges). In severely hypertensive subjects (i.e., diastolic pressure above 110 mm Hg), it is advisable to avoid anesthetics with a vasoconstrictor. If diastolic pressure is below 110, a vasoconstrictor is advisable to maintain deep anesthesia and to avoid endogenous catecholamine release as a consequence of loss of pain control. An aspiration syringe should be used, and the anesthetic should not be injected intravascularly. Extreme caution should be taken with patients who have known pseudocholinesterase deficiency (an enzyme that catabolizes procaine and its congeners).

INTERACTIONS:
1. alcohol—central nervous system and respiratory depression
2. antidepressants—central nervous system and respiratory depression
3. antiarrhythmic drugs—cardiac depression
4. antimyasthenics—antagonize antimyasthenic effects
5. beta-blockers—prolonged anesthetic effects

VASOCONSTRICTOR INTERACTIONS:
1. inhalation anesthetics—increased risk for arrhythmia
2. beta-blockers—hypertension
3. phenothiazines—hypotension
4. tricyclic antidepressants—tachycardia, systolic hypertension

INHALATION SEDATION

NITROUS OXIDE

ADVERSE EFFECTS: When used at 85% with 15% oxygen at the early induction phase followed by maintenance at 70% concentration with 30% oxygen, the adverse affects are minimal, with stage I analgesia being obtained. Toxic effects may occur at higher concentrations simply because oxygenation is inadequate. Postanalgesia diffusion hypoxia is a side effect that can be overcome by administration of pure oxygen for 3 to 5 minutes after analgesia. Pernicious anemia can occur with prolonged or consecutive administration of nitrous oxide because of its oxidation of cobalt in vitamin B_{12}.

CAUTIONS: Prescribe with care or do not use if the patient is taking other medications that are central nervous system depressants. Do not use under hyperbaric conditions, since convulsions may occur.

INTERACTIONS:
1. analgesics—accentuated analgesia
2. sedatives—accentuated analgesia

INTRAVENOUS SEDATION

METHOHEXITAL, SECOBARBITOL, THIOPENTAL, THIAMYLAL (Brevital, Seconal): short-term sedation for oral surgical procedures, usually used in conjunction with analgesics

ADVERSE EFFECTS: respiratory depression, laryngospasm, post-treatment hangover, depression, confusion, diarrhea, nausea; cardiac depression with hypotension in patients with cardiovascular disease

CAUTIONS: Prescribe with care or do not use if the patient is pregnant or allergic, or has porphyria, asthma, anemia, epilepsy, liver disease, or renal disease. In hypovolemic or septic patients, cardiac failure may occur during induction.

INTERACTIONS:
1. anticoagulants—decreased anticoagulation effect
2. anticonvulsants—altered seizures
3. antidepressants—increased sedation, counteracted antidepressant effect
4. antihistamines—marked sedation
5. aspirin—decreased analgesia
6. beta-blockers—decreased β-adrenergic effect
7. carbamazepine—decreased pain relief in trigeminal neuralgia
8. carteolol—increased sedation
9. clozapine—central nervous system toxicity
10. contraceptives—decreased contraceptive effect
11. divalproex—marked sedation
12. doxycycline—decreased antimicrobial effect
13. griseofulvin—decreased antifungal effect
14. hypoglycemics—increased sedation
15. monoamine oxidase inhibitors—increased sedation
16. narcotics—increased sedation
17. sedatives—marked sedation

BENZODIAZEPINES (Diazepam, Midazolam, Valium, Versed): diminish the anxiety component of surgical procedures

ADVERSE EFFECTS: Excitation or delirium in selected patients at therapeutic dosage. Euphoria can last 6 hours after administration of 5 to 10 mg. Slight cardiovascular and respiratory depression occurs.

CAUTIONS: Prescribe with care or do not use if the patient is hypotensive or suffers from obstructive pulmonary disease. Drug interactions with other analgesics, sedatives, and central nervous system depressants should be noted. Caution must be taken with patients suspected of drug or alcohol abuse.

INTERACTIONS:
1. anticonvulsants—alterations in seizure severity
2. antidepressants—increased sedation
3. antihypertensive agents—significant hypotensive effect
4. clozapine—severe central nervous system toxicity
5. contraceptives—increased sedation
6. disulfiram—increased sedation
7. antibiotics (erythromycin, ketoconazole)—increased sedation
8. L-dopa—decreased levodopa effect
9. monoamine oxidase inhibitors—severe side effects, convulsions
10. narcotics—increased sedation
11. tranquilizers—increased sedation
12. nizatidine—toxic effect of benzodiazepine

13. probenecid—increased sedation
14. zidovudine—bone marrow toxicity

KETAMINE: dissociative anesthesia for dental and oral surgery

ADVERSE EFFECTS: Slow nystagmus and myospasm in some patients. Respiratory depression, loss of laryngeal reflexes, hypertension, and increased intracranial pressure may occur during rapid infusion or high doses. Hypersalivation is also a complication and can be minimized by administration of antimuscarinic drugs. The cardiovascular stimulatory effects can be minimized or abrogated by addition of a benzodiazepine. Mental stress or anxiety may follow as a result of hallucinogenic effects, and some patients report recurring "flashbacks." Diazepam also minimizes these psychologic complications.

CAUTIONS: Prescribe with care or do not use if the patient has a history of allergies. Ketamine should be avoided in patients with cardiovascular disease, cranial trauma, glaucoma, hyperthyroidism, or schizophrenia.

INTERACTIONS
1. aminophylline—possible risk for seizures
2. benzodiazepines—increased ketamine effect, reduced cardiovascular side effects
3. droperidol—reduced cardiovascular side effects of ketamine
4. inhalation anesthetics—hypertension, decreased cardiac output
5. narcotics—increased risk for post-treatment hallucination
6. thyroxine—severe tachycardia, hypertension

INTRAMUSCULAR INJECTABLES

BOTULINUM TOXIN TYPE A (Botox): intramuscular injection for dystonia or persistent muscle-twitching of facial or masticatory muscles.

ADVERSE EFFECTS: muscle paralysis, which may become irreversible

CAUTIONS: Administer with care or do not use if the patient has a history of allergies. Because of toxicity, this drug should be used only in refractory spasms. The injection foci should be monitored by electromyography.

INTERACTIONS: none known.

TRIAMCINOLONE INJECTABLE (Aristocort, Aristospan, Kenalog): intralesion injection for bullous diseases, noninfectious granulomatous lesions, temporomandibular joint arthritis

ADVERSE EFFECTS: Immunosuppression is possible if the drug is used over a prolonged period. Single pulse injection raises blood levels only temporarily. Transiant headache, nausea, or vomiting is possible.

CAUTIONS: Administer with care or do not use if the patient has a history of allergy to triamcinolone or is pregnant. Aspiration prior to injection must be undertaken to ensure that the medication does not enter vessels.

INTERACTIONS: Steroids may interact with many other drugs when used on a steady basis. Local tissue injections are usually not of concern when the patient it taking other medications. The following interactions should, however, be noted:

1. anticholinergic agents—induction of glaucoma
2. anticoagulants—decreased anticoagulant effect
3. aspirin—increased steroidal effect
4. hypoglycemic agents—decreased hypoglycemic effect
5. thiazide diuretics—potassium depletion

SODIUM TETRADECYL SULFATE INJECTION (Sotradecol): sclerosis of varices and Kaposi's sarcoma

ADVERSE EFFECTS: Tissue necrosis can become widespread if drug is injected injudiciously. The drug can cause severe eye irritation. Postinjection pain is variable and can be severe in some patients. Prescription of an analgesic for postoperative pain is advisable.

CAUTIONS: Administer with care or do not use if the patient is allergic or pregnant. For first administration, only a minute amount should be injected, and the patient should be observed for a number of hours. If no adverse reactions occur, additional treatments can be administered.

INTERACTIONS: none known.

VINCA ALKALOIDS (vincristine, sulfate, Oncovin, vinblastine sulfate, Velban): used as a local antitumor injectable for treating Kaposi's sarcoma

ADVERSE EFFECTS: Intralesional injection is not associated with significant adverse effects such as may be encountered with intravenous administration. Lesion injection site is often painful. Vinca alkaloids are fatal if administered intrathecally. Bone marrow suppression with agranulocytopenia, anemia, or thrombocytopenia is possible. Alopecia, corneal irritation on contact, constipation, hypertension, bronchospasms, and aspermia in men may all occur.

CAUTIONS: Administer with care or do not use if the patient has a history of allergies. Use great care in patients with hematologic depression, cardiovascular disease, or chronic obstructive pulmonary disease.

INTERACTIONS:

1. antineoplastic drugs—increased bone marrow suppression
2. phenytoin—decreased antiseizure effect
3. steroids—amenorrhea

GINGIVAL DISPLACEMENT RETRACTION CORD

IMPREGNATED COTTON CORD (Hemodent): zinc and aluminum salt astringents, racemic epinephrine (1 mg per inch of cord)

ADVERSE EFFECTS: For string with epinephrine, tachycardia is possible in patients with hypertension or who are taking vasoactive medications. Aluminum and zinc strings are not known to cause adverse effects.

CAUTIONS: Do not use string with epinephrine in patients with a history of cardiovascular or renal disease.

INTERACTIONS (epinephrine-soaked cord):
1. inhalation anesthetics—increased risk for arrhythmia
2. beta-blockers—hypertension
3. phenothiazines—hypotension
4. tricyclic antidepressants—tachycardia, systolic hypertension

BIBLIOGRAPHY

Journals

Adams LE, Hess EV: Drug related lupus: Incidence, mechanisms and clinical implications. Drug Safety 6:431–449, 1991.

Adler-Storthz K, Newland JR, Tessin BA, et al: Identification of human papillomavirus types in oral verruca vulgaris. J Oral Pathol 15:230–235, 1986.

Adriani J, Campbell B: Fatalities following the topical application of local anesthetics to mucous membranes. JAMA 162:1527–1530, 1956.

Albright GA: Cardiac arrest following regional anesthesia with etidocaine or bupivacaine. Anesthesiology 51:285–287, 1979.

Allen CM, Beck FM: Strain-related differences in pathogenicity of *Candida albicans* for oral mucosa. J Infect Dis 147:1036–1040, 1983.

Allen CM, Blozis GG: Oral mucosal reactions to cinnamon-flavored chewing gum. J Am Dent Assoc 116:664–667, 1988.

Almeida ODP, Scully C: Oral lesions in the systemic mycoses. Curr Opin Dent 1:423–428, 1991.

Amess JAL, Burman JF, Rees GM, et al: Megaloblastic haematopoiesis in patients receiving nitrous oxide. Lancet 2:339–342, 1978.

Arendorf TM, Walker DM: The prevalence and intra-oral distribution of *Candida albicans* in man. Arch Oral Biol 25:1–10, 1980.

Arora S, Aldrete JA: Investigation of possible allergy to local anesthetic drugs: Correlation of intradermal with intramuscular injections. Anesth Rev 3:13–16, 1976.

Barrett AP: Oral changes as initial diagnostic indicators in acute leukemia. J Oral Med 41:234, 1986.

Boakes AJ, Lawrence DR, Lovel DW, et al: Adverse reactions to local anaesthetic/vasoconstrictor preparations. Br Dent J 133:137, 1972.

Bodey GP: Azole antifungal agents. Clin Infect Dis 14:S161–S169, 1992.

Bolewska J, Holmstrup P, Moller-Madsen B, et al: Amalgam associated mercury accumulations in normal oral mucosa, oral mucosal lesions of lichen planus and contact lesions associated with amalgam. J Oral Pathol Med 15:39–42, 1990.

Butt GM: Drug-induced xerostomia. J Can Dent Assoc 57:391–393, 1991.

Caranasos GJ, May FE, Stewart RB, Cluff LE: Drug associated deaths in hospital inpatients. Arch Intern Med 136:872, 1976.

Cawson RA: Denture sore mouth and angular cheilitis: Oral candidiasis in adults. Br Dent J 115:441–449, 1963.

Celesia GG, Chen RC, Bamforth, BJ: Effects of ketamine in epilepsy. Neurology 25:169–172, 1975.

Chan HL, Stern RS, Arndt KA, et al: The incidence of erythema multiforme, Stevens-Johnson syndrome, and toxic epidermal necrolysis: A population-based study with particular reference to reactions caused by drugs among outpatients. Arch Dermatol 126:43–47, 1990.

Cooper SA, Needle SE, Kruger GO: Comparative analgesic potency of aspirin and ibuprofen. J Oral Surg 35:898–903, 1977.

Council on Dental Therapeutics: Emergency kits. J Am Dent Assoc 87:909, 1973.

Council on Dental Therapeutics: Management of dental problems in patients with cardiovascular disease. American Dental Association and American Heart Association Joint Report. J Am Dent Assoc 68:333–342, 1964.

Crawford JS, Lewis M: Nitrous oxide in early human pregnancy. Anaesthesia 41:900–905, 1986.

Dajani AS, Bisno AL, Chung KJ, et al: Prevention of bacterial endocarditis: Recommendations by the American Heart Association. JAMA 264:2919–2922, 1990.

deShazo RD, Nelson HS: An approach to the patient with a history of local anesthetic hypersensitivity: Experience with 90 patients. J Allergy Clin Immunol 63:387–394; 1979.

Desjardins PJ: The top 20 prescription drugs and how they affect your dental practice. Compendium 13:740–756, 1992.

Dhunér K-G: Frequency of general side reactions after regional anaesthesia with mepivacaine with and without vasoconstrictors. Acta Anaesthesiol Scand (Suppl) 48:23–43, 1972.

Dougherty RJ: Propoxyphene overdose deaths. JAMA 235:2716, 1976.

Downs JR: Atypical cholinesterase activity: Its importance in dentistry. J Oral Surg 24:256, 1966.

Dreizen S, Bodey GP, Valdivieso M: Chemotherapy-associated oral infections in adults with solid tumors. Oral Surg Oral Med Oral Pathol 55:113, 1983.

Dreizen S, Brown LR, Handler SH, et al: Radiation-induced xerostomia in cancer patients. Cancer 38:273, 1976.

Duncan WK, Pruhs RH, Ashrafi MH, and Post AC: Chloral hydrate and other drugs used in sedating young children: A survey of American Academy of Pedodontics Diplomates. Pediatr Dent 5:252–256, 1983.

Eisenberg E, Krutchkoff DJ: Lichenoid lesions of the oral mucosa: Diagnostic criteria and their importance in the alleged relationship to oral cancer. Oral Surg Oral Med Oral Pathol 73:699–704, 1992.

Epstein JB, Scully C: Intralesional vinblastine for oral Kaposi's sarcoma in HIV infection. Lancet 2:1100–1101, 1989.

Epstein JB, Scully C: Herpes simplex in immunocompromised patients: Growing evidence of drug resistance. Oral Surg Oral Med Oral Pathol 72:47–50, 1991.

Eisen D, Ellis CN, Duell EA, et al: Effect of topical cyclosporine rinse on oral lichen planus: A double-blind analysis. N Engl J Med 323:290–294, 1990.

Eversole LR: Immunopathology of oral mucosal ulcerative, desquamative, and bullous diseases. Oral Surg Oral Med Oral Pathol 77:555–571, 1994.

Eversole LR: Inflammatory diseases of the mucous membranes. Part 1. Viral and fungal infections. Part. 2 Immunopathologic, ulcerative and desquamative diseases. J Calif Dent Assoc 22:52–57, 1994.

Eversole LR, Laipis PJ, Merrell P, Choi E: Demonstration of human papillomavirus DNA in oral condyloma acuminatum. J Oral Pathol Med 16:266–272, 1987.

Eversole LR, Leider AS, Jacobsen PC, Shaber EP: Oral Kaposi's sarcoma associated with acquired immunodeficiency syndrome among homosexual males. J Am Dent Assoc 107:248–253, 1983.

Eversole LR, Stone CE, Beckman AM: Detection of EBV and HPV-DNA sequences in oral "hairy" leukoplakia by in-situ hybridization. J Med Virol 26:271–277, 1988.

Ficarra G, Berson AM, Silverman S, et al: Kaposi's sarcoma of the oral cavity: A study of 134 patients with a review of the pathogenesis, epidemiology, clinical aspects and treatment. Oral Surg Oral Med Oral Pathol 66:543–550, 1988.

Forbes JA, Claderazzo JP, Bowser MW, et al: A 12-hour evaluation of the analgesic efficacy of diflunisal, aspirin and placebo in postoperative dental pain. J Clin Pharmacol 22:89–96, 1982.

Glauda NM, Henefer EP, Supur S: Nonfatal anaphylaxis caused by penicillin: Report of case. J Am Dent Assoc 90:159, 1975.

Glick M, Cohen SG, Cheney RT, et al: Oral manifestations of disseminated *Cryptococcus neoformans* in a patient with acquired immunodeficiency syndrome. Oral Surg Oral Med Oral Pathol 64:454–459, 1987.

Gogerty JH, Strand HA, Ogilvie AL, Dille JM: Vasopressor effects of topical epinephrine in certain dental procedures. Oral Surg Oral Med Oral Pathol, 10:614–622, 1957.

Goodson JM, Moore PA: Life-threatening reaction after pedodontic sedation: An assessment of narcotic, local anesthetic, and antiemetic drug interaction. J Am Dent Assoc 107:239–245, 1983.

Granoff DM, McDaniel DB, Barkowf SP: Cardiorespiratory arrest following aspiration of chloral hydrate. Am J Dis Child 122:170–171, 1971.

Greaves M, Lawlor F: Angioedema: manifestations and management. J Am Acad Dermatol 25:155–165, 1991.

Green JA, Spruance SL, Wenerstrom G, Pipkorn MW: Post-herpetic erythema multiforme prevented with prophylactic oral acyclovir. Ann Intern Med 102:632–633, 1985.

Green TL, Eversole LR: Oral lymphomas in HIV-infected patients: Association with Epstein-Barr virus DNA. Oral Surg 67:437–442, 1989.

Greenberg MS, Friedman H, Cohen SG, et al: A comparative study of herpes simplex infections in renal transplant and leukemic patients. J Infect Dis 156:280–287, 1987.

Greenblatt DJ, Koch-Weser J: Adverse reactions to intravenous diazepam: A report from the Boston Collaborative Drug Surveillance Program. Am J Med Sci 266:261, 1973.

Greenspan D, Greenspan JS: Oral mucosal manifestations of AIDS. Dermatol Clin 5:733–737, 1987.

Greenspan D, Greenspan JS, DeSouza YG, et al: Oral "hairy" leukoplakia in male homosexuals: Evidence of association with both papillomavirus and a herpes-group virus. Lancet 2:831–834, 1984.

Greer R, Eversole LR: Detection of HPV genomic DNA in oral epithelial dysplasias, smokeless tobacco-associated leukoplakias and epithelial malignancies. J Oral Maxillofac Surg 48:1201–1205, 1990.

Grzelewska-Rzymowska I, Szmidt M, Rozniecki J: Urticaria/angioedema-type sensitivity to aspirin and other non-steroidal anti-inflammatory drugs: Diagnostic value of anamnesis and challenge test with acetylsalicylic acid. J Invest Allergol Clin Immunol 2:191–195, 1992.

Hedner T, Samuelsson O, Lindholm AL, Wiholm BE: Precipitation of angioedema by antihypertensive drugs. J Hypertens 9:S360–S361, 1991.

Hersh EV, Helpin ML, Evans OB: Local anesthetic mortality: Report of case. ASDC J Dent Child 58:489–491, 1991.

Holmstrup P, Thorn JJ, Rindum J, Pindborg JJ: Malignant development of lichen planus–affected oral mucosa. J Oral Pathol 17:219–225, 1988.

Holroyd SV, Watts DT, Welch JT.: The use of epinephrine in local anesthetics for dental patients with cardiovascular disease: A review of the literature. J Oral Surg 18:492, 1960.

Houpt MI, Koenigsberg SR, Weiss NJ, Desjardins PJ: Comparison of chloral hydrate with and without promethazine in the sedation of young children. Pediatr Dent 7:41–46, 1985.

Houston JB, Appleby RC, DeCountet L, et al: Effect of r-epinephrine impregnated retraction cord on the cardiovascular system. J Prosthet Dent 24:373, 1970.

Huston DP, Bressler RB: Urticaria and angioedema. Med Clin North Am 76:805–840, 1992.

Isaksson M, Bruze M, Bjorkner B, Niklasson B: Contact allergy to Duraphat. Scand J Dent Res 101:49–51, 1993.

Israili ZH, Hall WD: Cough and angioneurotic edema associated with angiotensin-converting enzyme inhibitor therapy: A review of the literature and pathophysiology. Ann Intern Med 117:234–242, 1992.

Jastak JT, Yageila JA: Vasoconstrictors and local anesthesia: A review and rationale for use. J Am Dent Assoc 107:623–630, 1983.

Korman NJ, Eyre RW, Zone J, Stanley JR: Drug-induced pemphigus: Autoantibodies directed against the pemphigus antigen complexes are present in penicillamine and captopril-induced pemphigus. J Invest Dermatol 96:273–276, 1991.

Laeijendecker R, Van Joost T: Oral manifestations of gold allergy. J Am Acad Dermatol 30:205–209, 1994.

Lamey PJ, Rees TD, Binnie WH, Rankin KV: Mucous membrane pemphigoid: Treatment experience at two institutions. Oral Surg Oral Med Oral Pathol 74:50–53, 1992.

Lamey PJ, Rees TD, Binnie WH, et al: Oral presentation of pemphigus vulgaris and its response to systemic steroid therapy. Oral Surg Oral Med Oral Pathol 74:54–57, 1992.

Langford A, Kunze R, Timm H, et al: Cytomegalovirus associated oral ulcerations in HIV-infected patients. J Oral Pathol Med 19:71–76, 1990.

Laskaris G, Satriano RA: Drug-induced blistering oral lesions. Clin Dermatol 11:545–550, 1993.

Lauven PM: Pharmacology of drugs for conscious sedation. Scand J Gastroenterol 179(Suppl):1–6, 1990.

Layzer RB, Fishman RA, Schafer JA: Neuropathy following abuse of nitrous oxide. Neurology 28:504–506, 1978.

Levine MJ, Aguirre A, Hatton MN, et al: Artificial salivas: Present and future. J Dent Res 66:693, 1987.

Lind PO: Oral lichenoid reactions related to composite restorations: Preliminary report. Acta Odontol Scand 54:53–55, 1988.

Loning T, Ikenberg H, Becker J, et al: Analysis of oral papillomas, leukoplakias, and invasive carcinomas for human papillomavirus type related DNA. J Invest Dermatol 84:417–420, 1985.

Loning T, Reichart P, Staquet MJ, et al: Occurrence of papillomavirus structural antigens in oral papillomas and leukoplakias. J Oral Pathol Med 13:155–165, 1984.

Lozada-Nur F, Huang MZ, Zhou GA: Open preliminary clinical trial of clobetasol propionate ointment in adhesive paste for treatment of chronic oral vesiculoerosive diseases. Oral Surg Oral Med Oral Pathol 71:283–287, 1991.

Lozada-Nur F, Shillitoe EJ: Erythema multiforme and herpes simplex virus. J Dent Res 64:930, 1985.

McCarthy FM, Malamed SF: Physical evaluation system to determine medical risk and indicated dental therapy modifications. J Am Dent Assoc 99:181–184, 1979.

Miescher PA: Drug induced thrombocytopenia. Semin Hematol 10:311, 1973.

Miller RL, Gould AR, Bernstein ML: Cinnamon-induced stomatitis venenata: Clinical and characteristic histopathologic features. Oral Surg Oral Med Oral Pathol 73:708–716, 1992.

Mosteller JH: The ability of a prednisolone solution to eliminate pulpal inflammation. J Prosthet Dent 13:754–760, 1963.

Munoz RJ: The cardiovascular effects of anxiety and r-epinephrine retraction cord in routine fixed prosthodontic procedures. J Calif Dent Assoc 46:10, 1970.

Newcomb GM: Contraindications to the use of catecholamine vasoconstrictors in dental local analgesics. N Z Dent J 69:25–30, 1973.

Nunn JF, Sharer NM: Megaloblastic haemopoiesis after multiple short-term exposure to nitrous oxide. Lancet 1:1379–1381, 1982.

Oda D, MacDougall L, Fritsche T, Worthington P: Oral histoplasmosis as a presenting disease in acquired immunodeficiency syndrome. Oral Surg Oral Med Oral Pathol 70:631–636, 1990.

Pague WL, Harrison JD: Absorption of epinephrine during tissue retraction. J Prosthet Dent 18:242, 1967.

Pemberton M, Yeoman CM, Clark A, et al: Allergy to octyl gallate causing stomatitis. Br Dent J 175:106–108, 1993.

Persson G: General side effects of local dental anesthesia with special reference to catecholamines as vasoconstrictors and to the effect of some premedicants. Acta Odont Scand 53(Suppl):1–60, 1969.

Pérusse R, Goulet J-P, Turcotte J-Y: Contraindications to vasoconstrictors in dentistry. Oral Surg Oral Med Oral Pathol 74:679–691, 1992.

Phatak NM, Lang RL: Systemic hemodynamic effects of r-epinephrine gingival retraction cord in clinic patients. J Oral Ther Pharmacol 2:393, 1966.

Rehorst ED, DeGroot GW: Preoperative management of glucocorticoid dependent pedodontic patients. J Am Dent Assoc 93:809, 1976.

Robertson WD, Wray D: Ingestion of medication among patients with oral keratoses including lichen planus. Oral Surg Oral Med Oral Pathol 74:183–185, 1992.

Samaranayake LP, Scully C: Oral candidosis in HIV infection. Lancet 2:1491–1492, 1989.

Scoggins RB, Kliman B: Percutaneous absorption of corticosteroids. J Clin Endocrinol 25:11, 1965.

Scully C: Orofacial herpes simplex virus infections: Current concepts on the epidemiology, pathogenesis and treatment and disorders in which the virus may be implicated. Oral Surg Oral Med Oral Pathol 68:701–710, 1989.

Scully C, Almeida ODP: Orofacial manifestations of the systemic mycoses. J Oral Pathol Med 21:289–294, 1992.

Scully C, Porter SR: Orofacial manifestations in HIV infection. Lancet 1:976–977, 1988.

Seldin HM: Survey of anesthetic fatalities in oral surgery and a review of the etiological factors in anesthetic deaths. J Am Dent Soc Anesthesiol 5:5–12, 1958.

Silverman S Jr, Gorsky M, Losada-Nur F, Giannotti K: A prospective study of findings and management in 214 patients with oral lichen planus. Oral Surg Oral Med Oral Pathol 72:665–670, 1991.

Spear PW, Protass LM: Barbiturate poisoning: An endemic disease. Med Clin North Am 57:1471, 1973.

Spruance SL: Pathogenesis of herpes simplex labialis: Excretion of virus in the oral cavity. J Clin Microbiol 19:675–679, 1984.

Staerkjaer L, Menne T: Nickel allergy and orthodontic treatment. Eur J Orthodont 12:284–289, 1990.

Stampien TM, Schwartz RA: Erythema multiforme. Am Family Physician 46:1171–1176, 1992.

Staretz LR, DeBoom GW: Multiple oral and skin lesions occurring after treatment with penicillin. J Am Dent Assoc 121:436–437, 1990.

Streeten DHP: Corticosteroid therapy. II. Complications and therapeutic indications, JAMA 232:1046, 1975.

Strom BL, Carson JL, Halpern AC, et al: A population-based study of Stevens Johnson syndrome. Incidence and antecedent drug exposures. Arch Dermatol 127:831–838, 1991.

Syrjanen KJ: Epidemiology of human papillomavirus (HPV) infections and their associations with genital squamous cell cancer. APMIS 97:957–970, 1989.

Tekavec MM: Nitrous oxide sedation with auditory modification. Anesth Progr 23:181–186, 1976.

Thompson WM, Brown RH, Williams SM: Medication and perception of dry mouth in a population of institutionalized elderly people. N Z Med J 106:219–221, 1993.

Thorn JJ, Holmstrup P, Rindum J, Pindborg JJ: Course of various clinical forms of oral lichen planus: A prospective follow-up study of 611 patients. J Oral Pathol 17:213–218, 1988.

Toller PA: Use and misuse of intra-articular corticosteroids in treatment of temporomandibular joint pain. Proc R Soc Med 70:461–463, 1977.

van Loon LA, Bos JD, Davidson CL: Clinical evaluation of fifty-six patients referred with symptoms tentatively related to allergic contact stomatitis. Oral Surg Oral Med Oral Pathol 74:572–575, 1992.

Vernale CA: Cardiovascular responses to local dental anesthesia with epinephrine in normotensive and hypertensive subjects. Oral Surg Oral Med Oral Pathol 13:942–952, 1960.

Verrill PJ: Adverse reactions to local anesthetics and vasoconstrictor drugs. Practitioner 214:380–387, 1975.

Watts SL, Brewer EE, Fry TL: Human papillomavirus DNA types in squamous cell carcinomas of the head and neck. Oral Surg Oral Med Oral Pathol 71:701–707, 1991.

Williams DM: Vesiculobullous mucocutaneous disease: Pemphigus vulgaris. J Oral Pathol Med 18:544–553, 1989.

Williams DM: Vesiculo-bullous mucocutaneous disease: Benign mucous membrane and bullous pemphigoid. J Oral Pathol Med 19:16–23, 1990.

Wood M: Pharmacokinetic drug interactions in anaesthetic practice. Clin Pharmacokinet 21:285–307, 1991.

Yagiela JA: Intravascular lidocaine toxicity: Influence of epinephrine and route of administration. Anesth Progr 32:57–61, 1985.

Yagiela JA: Death in a cardiac patient after local anesthesia with epinephrine. Orofacial Pain Management 1:6, 1991.

Yung RL, Richardson BC: Drug-induced lupus. Rheum Dis Clin North Am 20:61–86, 1994.

Zain RB: Oral lichenoid reactions during antimalarial prophylaxis with sulphadoxine-pyrimethamine combination. Southeast Asian J Trop Med Public Health 20:253–256, 1989.

Books

Allen GD: Dental Anesthesia and Analgesia. 3rd ed. Baltimore, Williams & Wilkins, 1984.

Batakis, JG: Tumors of the Head and Neck: Clinical and Pathological Considerations. Baltimore, Williams & Wilkins, 1974.

Eversole LR: Clinical Outline of Oral Pathology. 3rd ed. Philadelphia, Lea & Febiger, 1992.

Greenspan D, Greenspan JS, Pindborg JJ, Schoidt M: AIDS and the Dental Team. Copenhagen, Munksgaard, 1986.

Griffith HW: Complete Guide to Prescription and Non-Prescription Drugs. New York, Putnam Berkley, 1992.

Holroyd SV, Wynn RL: Clinical Pharmacology in Dental Practice. St. Louis, CV Mosby, 1983.

Little JW, Falace DA: Dental Management of the Medically Compromised Patient. St. Louis, CV Mosby, 1980.

Lynch MA (ed): Burkett's Oral Medicine: Diagnosis and Treatment. Philadelphia, JB Lippincott, 1984.

Malamed SF: Handbook of Medical Emergencies in the Dental Office. 3rd ed. St. Louis, CV Mosby, 1982.

Neidle EA, Yagiela JA: Pharmacology and Therapeutics for Dentistry. 3rd ed. St. Louis, CV Mosby, 1989.

Regezi JA, Sciubba J: Oral Pathology: Clinical–Pathologic Correlations. Philadelphia, WB Saunders, 1993.

Robinson HBG, Miller AS: Color Atlas of Oral Pathology. Philadelphia, JB Lippincott, 1990.

Rondanelli R: Clinical Pharmacology of Drug Interactions. Padova, Italy, Piccin Nuova Libraria, 1988.

Samaranayake LP, MacFarlane TW (eds): Oral Candidosis. London, Butterworths, 1990.

Shinn AF (ed): Evaluations of Drug Interactions. New York, Macmillan, 1988.

Silverman S: Color Atlas of Oral Manifestations of Aids. Toronto, Decker, 1989.

Winkler JR, Grassi M, Murray PA: Clinical description and etiology of HIV-associated periodontal diseases. In: Robertson PB, Greenspan JS (eds): Oral Manifestations of AIDS. Littleton, MA, PSG, 1988, pp 49–70.

Yagiela J: Local anesthetics. In: Dionne RA, Phero JC (eds): Management of Pain and Anxiety in Dental Practice. New York, Elsevier, 1991, Chap 7, pp 109–134.

INDEX

Note: Page numbers in *italics* refer to illustrations.